Control irritable bowel syndrome for life

IBS
FOOD, FACTS
& RECIPES

TRACY PARKER & SARA LEWIS

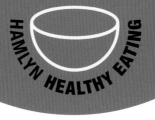

HAMLYN HEALTHY EATING

CAUTIONS

People with known nut allergies should avoid recipes containing nuts or nut derivatives, and vulnerable people should avoid dishes containing raw or lightly cooked eggs.

If you are avoiding wheat and gluten, double-check the ingredients list on items, such as mustard and stock cubes, before use. In addition, some brands of cornflour contain wheat flour to keep it free flowing, so read the ingredients list carefully if you are avoiding gluten.

Many of the recipes can be adapted for either a high- or low-fibre diet by using brown or white rice, pasta and flour or by using different combinations of vegetables, and recipes can be adapted for milk-free diets by the inclusion of soya milk and yogurt instead of cows' milk, yogurt and fromage frais.

Part of the nutritional information provided is sodium. These amounts only cover added salt when a specific amount is stated in the recipes.

Nutritional analysis is provided for each recipe and given per serving.

This book is not intended to replace medical care under the direct supervision of a qualified doctor. Before embarking on any changes in your health regime, consult your doctor. While the advice and information are believed to be accurate and true at the time of going to press, neither the author nor the publisher can accept legal responsibility or liability for any errors or omissions that may have been made.

Ovens should be preheated to the specific temperature. If using a fan-assisted oven, follow the manufacturer's instructions for adjusting the time and temperature. Grills should also be preheated.

Both metric and imperial measurements are given for the recipes. Use one set of measurements only, not a mixture of both.

An Hachette UK company
www.hachette.co.uk

First published in Great Britain in 2007 by
Hamlyn, a division of Octopus Publishing Group Limited
Endeavour House, 189 Shaftesbury Avenue,
London WC2H 8JY
www.octopusbooks.co.uk

This edition published in 2015

Copyright © Octopus Publishing Group Limited 2007, 2015

Tracy Parker and Sara Lewis assert the moral right to be identified as the authors of this work.

ISBN 978-0600-63033-3

A CIP catalogue record for this book is available from the British Library

Printed and bound in China

10 9 8 7 6 5 4 3 2 1

contents

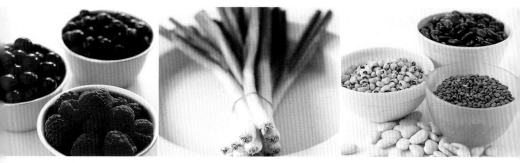

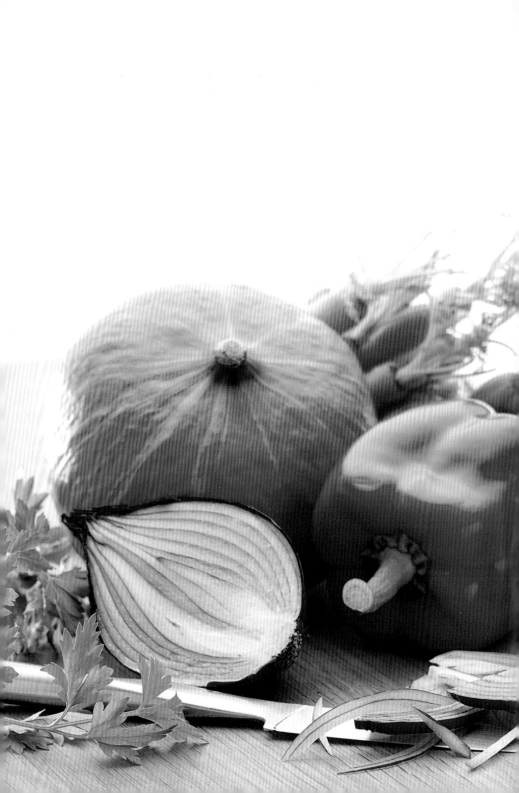

introduction

Irritable Bowel Syndrome (IBS) is a common bowel condition, which is said to affect as many as one in five of the adult populations of Britain and the USA. People of any age can suffer with IBS, including children, but the most common age range affected is 20–40 years, and women are twice as likely to report symptoms of IBS than men.

The cause of IBS is not known, although there are many factors involved, and often the symptoms are the result of a combination of factors rather than just one. At present, there is no single cure for IBS, but there are lots of different ways to manage it, and tailoring your diet to deal with the symptoms you experience is a good place to start. It is important to remember, however, that dietary changes will not help everyone, and if your symptoms persist you should seek medical advice.

what is Irritable Bowel Syndrome?

'Self-diagnosis of IBS is not advisable. Before a diagnosis is made it is important that a doctor carries out appropriate examinations and investigations.'

OTHER CONDITIONS WITH SIMILAR SYMPTOMS

- Diverticulitis
- Gallstones
- Bile salt malabsorption
- Microscopic colitis
- Chronic fatigue syndrome
- Coeliac disease
- Inflammatory bowel disease (Crohn's disease or ulcerative colitis)
- Bowel cancer

Irritable Bowel Syndrome (IBS) is described as a functional bowel disorder by the medical profession. This means that no specific cause can be found for an individual's symptoms after medical investigations but that the bowel is functioning in an abnormal way.

Symptoms

The key symptoms for a diagnosis of IBS are that the person should have suffered abdominal pain or discomfort for at least 12 weeks (this does not have to be consecutive weeks) during the last 12 months. In addition, two of the following three symptoms should also be present:

- ☐ Relief of pain or discomfort with passing a bowel motion (defecation)
- ☐ A change in the frequency of stools – an increase or decrease in bowel motions
- ☐ A change in the consistency of stools – looser or harder motions

Additional symptoms

There is a further group of symptoms that support the diagnosis of IBS, and two or more of these should be present on at least 25 per cent of occasions or days when IBS is suspected. These supportive symptoms are:

- ☐ Altered stool frequency: more than three bowel motions a day or fewer than three bowel movements a week
- ☐ Altered stool form: looser or more watery motions, or hard, lumpy or pellet-like motions
- ☐ Altered stool passage: straining to pass a motion or urgency or the feeling of not completely emptying the bowel (incomplete evacuation)

☐ Passing mucus with stools
☐ Abdominal bloating or distension

In addition to the above symptoms, many people with IBS often complain of flatulence (wind), rumbling noises in the bowel (borborygmi), indigestion or heartburn, nausea, headaches, persistent tiredness and an increased need to urinate. Women sometimes also find sexual intercourse painful.

Is it IBS?

Self-diagnosis of IBS is not advisable. Before a diagnosis is made it is important that a medical doctor carries out appropriate examinations and investigations. This is because there are several other, more serious bowel conditions that have similar symptoms to those of IBS. Further investigation may be necessary if any of the following are present:

☐ Recent, unexplained weight loss
☐ Rectal bleeding
☐ Anaemia
☐ Fever
☐ Start of symptoms over the age of 50 years
☐ Recurrent vomiting
☐ A family history of colon cancer, Crohn's disease, ulcerative colitis or coeliac disease

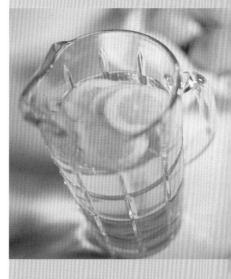

possible causes of IBS

'It is not known if stress causes IBS in the first place, but the symptoms of IBS can certainly make people anxious.'

There are many different theories about the causes of IBS, and there are almost as many different ideas about how to treat it. The main causes are believed to be a bout of bacterial gastroenteritis, the use of antibiotics, stress and anxiety and other psychological reasons, abnormal gut motility and hypersensitivity of the gut, the menstrual cycle in women and diet.

Post-infective IBS
Some people with IBS can link the start of their symptoms to having had a bowel infection or gastroenteritis, such as salmonella food poisoning. Research has shown that people who have had severe gastroenteritis are almost 12 times more likely to develop IBS than those who have not. It is not clear why this is the case, although changes to a person's normal gut bacteria have been suggested, as have slight changes to the bowel itself. This type of IBS is known as post-infective IBS.

Antibiotics
Everyone's large bowel contains billions of bacteria. The bacteria are of hundreds of different types, some of them beneficial to our health and others with the potential to cause ill health. In normal circumstances these bacteria live in a balance together and cause no problems to the individual. However, a course of antibiotics, prescribed to kill the bacteria causing a particular infection, can also kill the good bacteria in the bowel. This leads to an imbalance, which can result in symptoms such as diarrhoea, abdominal bloating, pain and flatulence.

Stress and anxiety

Many people find that stress or anxiety triggers their IBS, and some sufferers can link the start of their symptoms with times of change or upheaval in their life, such as leaving home, starting work, getting married or going to university. Other upsetting events include relationship problems, bereavement and physical or sexual abuse.

Stress has been shown to increase the speed at which waste is moved through the large bowel (colon), so leading to more frequent bowel motions. It also releases chemicals in the body that stimulate the colon, which leads to pain. It is not known if stress causes IBS in the first place, but the symptoms of IBS can certainly make people anxious, especially if their symptoms are frequent and unpleasant. Some people with IBS also have psychiatric illnesses.

Abnormal gut movement and hypersensitivity

Research has shown that in some people with IBS waste is moved through the gut more slowly or more quickly than normal. A slower movement may result in constipation, whereas a faster movement may lead to diarrhoea. There is also evidence that some people with IBS are more sensitive to discomfort in the bowel than people without IBS.

Research is being carried out into the ways in which the brain deals with pain or the anticipation of pain because there is some evidence that this does not work normally in IBS sufferers.

Menstrual cycle

IBS symptoms can be affected by the change in hormone levels that occur in the body over the menstrual cycle. Most women notice a change in their bowel motions during menstruation. It is not more common in IBS, but it may have more effect. As with some menstrual disorders, evening primrose oil may help with IBS symptoms.

'Exercise stimulates the body to produce feel good substances called endorphines, which help reduce stress.'

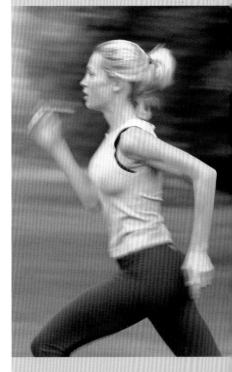

diet and IBS

The way we eat, what we eat and our meal patterns can all trigger the symptoms of IBS. Unfortunately, there is no one dietary change that will help everyone who is diagnosed with IBS. A change that will help one person may make the symptoms worse in another.

Meal patterns
It is important to have regular meals throughout the day. Missing meals and then snacking on high-fat, sugary foods or having one huge meal a day can lead to bloating, abdominal discomfort and wind.

How and what we eat
Eating quickly and rushing meals can lead to air being swallowed at the same time. This can result in belching or indigestion, and it can cause abdominal bloating and wind. Eating slumped over a computer keyboard or dashing around at the same time as eating can also cause problems. Always take time over your meals and sit up straight when you are eating.

Many foods have been identified as triggers to IBS symptoms, and these are considered in more detail on the following pages. However, simply adopting a balanced diet quite often helps people with IBS to control their symptoms.

Portion sizes
The bowel is made up of muscles that contract and relax one after another in sequence to push food through the digestive tract. A large meal can cause a stronger wave of muscle contraction, resulting in abdominal discomfort, indigestion and nausea. Keep to moderate portion sizes and healthy eating guidelines.

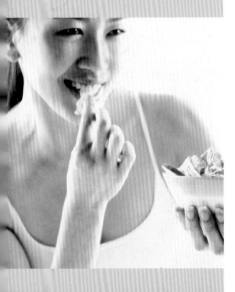

a balanced diet

A balanced diet is one that provides the body with all the nutrients it requires for health. In practice, this means choosing foods from the five food groups in the recommended amounts. The five food groups are: proteins, starchy foods, milk and dairy products, fruit and vegetables, and fats and sugars.

Protein

The body needs protein for growth and to repair cells. Protein-containing foods can be divided into animal proteins and vegetable proteins. Animal sources of protein are meat, including poultry and offal, fish and eggs; vegetable sources are beans, lentils and nuts. These foods are also good sources of iron, zinc, magnesium and B vitamins.

It is recommended that we include two servings of these foods a day. Try to choose leaner cuts of meat, trim away visible fat and remove the skin from poultry. You should also avoid frying meat to keep your fat intake down. This is recommended for general health, but fatty foods can also make IBS symptoms worse.

Starchy foods

Starchy foods are good sources of carbohydrates, which provide energy as well as B vitamins and fibre. Bread, pasta, rice, breakfast cereals and potatoes are good sources of starchy carbohydrates, and it is recommended that one-third of our daily diet should come from these foods – around 7–10 portions a day for women and 8–12 portions a day for men – so including a starchy food at every meal is important.

GUIDELINE PORTIONS OF PROTEIN FOODS

100 g (3½ oz) lean meat or poultry
100 g (3½ oz) oily fish
150 g (5 oz) white fish
2 eggs
4 tablespoons of cooked pulses or lentils

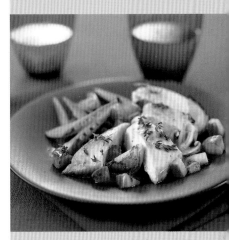

GUIDELINE PORTIONS OF STARCHY FOODS

1 slice of medium-cut bread
½ roll
½ pitta bread
1 small chapatti
2 egg-sized potatoes
2 heaped tablespoons of cooked rice or pasta
3 crispbreads or crackers
3 tablespoons of breakfast cereal
3 tablespoons of dry porridge oats

GUIDELINE PORTIONS OF MILK AND DAIRY PRODUCTS

40 g (1½ oz) cheese

200 ml (7 fl oz) milk

125 g (4 oz) yogurt

125 g (4 oz) fromage frais

200 ml (7 fl oz) calcium-enriched soya milk

200 ml (7 fl oz) calcium-enriched rice milk

125 g (4 oz) soya dessert or yogurt

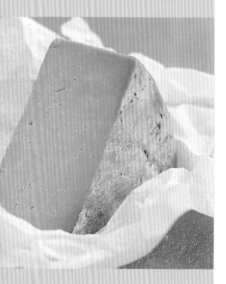

'It is recommended that no more than one-twelfth of our daily food intake comes from fats and sugars.'

Milk and dairy products

Milk and dairy products are an excellent source of calcium, as well as protein and vitamins A, B12 and D. Included in this group are milk, cheese, yogurt and fromage frais. Butter and cream are not included because they are high in fat and are therefore found in the fats and sugar group. It is recommended that we include three servings of these foods a day.

Fruit and vegetables

Fruit and vegetables are good sources of vitamin C, folate, carotenoids, potassium and fibre. All types of fruit and vegetable are included in this group except potatoes, which are classed as a starchy food. Fruit and vegetables can be fresh, frozen, tinned or dried. It is recommended that we have a minimum of five portions of these foods each day (see page 17).

Fats and sugars

Fatty and sugary foods tend to be high in calories and low in essential nutrients, and are often high in salt. Although it is fine to include them in small amounts in a varied diet, too much of them can lead to weight gain. It is recommended that only one-twelfth of our daily food intake comes from these foods. High-fat foods include butter, margarine, oils, fried foods, crisps and savoury snacks and pastry. High-sugar foods include sweets, chocolate, cakes, biscuits, soft drinks and drinks and ice cream.

How much fluid?

It is recommended that we have 8–10 cups of fluid a day, which is equivalent to 1.5–2 litres (2½–3½ pints). It is a myth that this fluid should be made up of just water. Any type of drink counts towards the recommended amount (except alcohol). Certain types of drinks, however, can trigger symptoms of IBS (see page 13).

Fluids

As much as 70 per cent of an adult's body weight is water. Throughout the day we lose water in our sweat, breath, urine and faeces, and if we do not replace the fluid we lose we suffer from dehydration, which leads to headaches, a lack of concentration, tiredness and dark-coloured urine. Continued inadequate intakes can lead to constipation and increase the risk of cystitis.

There are times when your body will need more fluid, such as when exercising, in a hot environment, if you have a temperature or if you have frequent diarrhoea or vomiting.

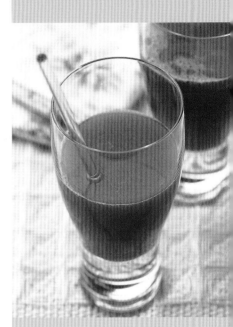

Caffeine As a stimulant caffeine gives us the kick-start we sometimes need. However, it also acts as an irritant to the bowel and can increase the need to urinate. Excessive amounts of caffeine can exacerbate the symptoms of IBS, so keep to a maximum of four or five caffeine-rich drinks a day and alternate them with caffeine-free drinks or water. Remember that some foods and pain-killing tablets contain caffeine too.

Alcohol Alcohol is also an irritant to the bowel and it can contribute to diarrhoea, abdominal discomfort and indigestion (heartburn). Ideally, keep within the recommended sensible limits for alcohol (14 units a week for women and 21 units a week for men) and have some alcohol-free days. Alcohol does help us to relax, and stress is linked with IBS, so a glass of wine at the end of a busy day can be helpful.

Fizzy drinks The gas in fizzy drinks can give abdominal bloating, belching and discomfort. Limit your intake of these drinks to one glass of 250–300 ml (8–10 fl oz) a day. These drinks include sparkling water, lemonade, cola, mixers added to spirits, soda water and sparkling fruit juice drinks.

CAFFEINE-RICH FOODS AND DRINKS

- Coffee, tea, hot chocolate, performance drinks, cola and chocolate

CAFFEINE-FREE DRINKS

- Decaffeinated coffee and tea, herbal and fruit teas, fruit juice, fruit squashes, still mineral water and flavoured still water, tapwater, milk and soya milk

ALCOHOL UNITS

For the purposes of assessing your intake, one unit of alcohol is:

300 ml (½ pint) standard-strength beer, lager or cider

1 small glass (125 ml or 4 fl oz) wine

1 glass of sherry

1 shot (25 ml or 1 fl oz) of spirits

dietary fibre

GOOD SOURCES OF SOLUBLE FIBRE:

- Oats, barley, pulses, seeds, fruit and vegetables

GOOD SOURCES OF INSOLUBLE FIBRE:

- Skins, peel and pips on fruit and vegetables, wheat, rye and nuts

SOURCES OF RESISTANT STARCH:

- Cooked potato, pasta and rice eaten cold or re-heated

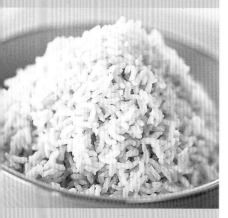

Dietary fibre, sometimes referred to as roughage, is part of plant foods that our bodies find difficult to digest. It is found in fruits, vegetables, cereals, pulses, nuts and seeds. It is part of the carbohydrate family, along with sugars and starches, and is known as complex carbohydrate or non-starch polysaccharide (NSP) in the scientific world.

Bacteria

Bacteria in the large intestine are able to break down fibre by a process called fermentation. This results in the production of gases, which are removed from the body as wind or are carried by the bloodstream to the lungs and expired on the breath. They also create substances called short chain fatty acids, which provide essential energy for the cells of the large intestine and also for the growth of the bacteria themselves.

Soluble and insoluble fibre

Fibre is divided into two types: soluble and insoluble fibre. Soluble fibre forms a gel-like substance in the intestine, and it has been shown to lower blood sugar and cholesterol levels.

Insoluble fibre absorbs water and helps provide bulky, easier-to-pass stools.

Resistant starch

Starch is found in foods such as potatoes, bread and rice and in some fruits. It was thought that all starch was digested in the small intestine, but it is now known that some starch is resistant to this process. It reaches the large intestine, where it is fermented by gut bacteria.

high and low fibre

IBS symptoms can be affected by the amount of fibre in your diet. Too little fibre can cause constipation and too much can cause bloating, discomfort and wind. It can also trigger diarrhoea. Altering the amount and type of fibre you eat can help control IBS symptoms.

High-fibre diets

A high-fibre diet may benefit people whose main symptom of IBS is constipation without abdominal bloating or wind.

It is important to increase the intake of both soluble and insoluble fibre and to have an adequate fluid intake – that is, 8–10 cups or 1.5–2 litres (2½–3½ pints) every day. Increase your intake of fibre gradually, over several days, because a sudden increase can give abdominal discomfort and wind. In addition, there is no benefit from having more than 32 g (about 1 oz) of fibre a day, and the recommended daily intake is 18 g (just over ½ oz).

Fibre supplements

Adding wheat bran to the diet to increase fibre intake is not recommended. Research has shown that it can make the symptoms of abdominal pain and bloating worse, and bran also interferes with the absorption of minerals, such as calcium, zinc and iron, from the diet.

Low-fibre diets

Healthy-eating guidelines suggest that we should increase our intake of fibre to decrease the risk of developing bowel cancer and diverticular disease. However, some people with IBS find that increasing

INCREASING FIBRE INTAKE

Among the best ways of increasing your intake of fibre are:

- Choosing wholemeal, granary or seeded breads
- Changing to brown rice or wholemeal pasta or mixing half white and half brown together
- Keeping the skins on vegetables and fruit
- Eating wholewheat breakfast cereals, such as Weetabix or bran flakes, or oat-based cereals, such as porridge
- Aiming to have at least five portions of fruit and vegetables every day
- Having seeds, nuts or dried fruit as snacks
- Adding pulses to stews and casseroles

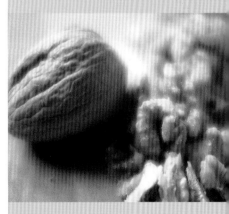

DECREASING FIBRE INTAKE

Among the best ways of decreasing your intake of fibre are:

- Changing to white bread and rolls
- Choosing baked products made with white flour, such as muffins, scones, crumpets and cake
- Having white pasta and rice and always eating it hot (cold pasta and rice are high in resistant starch)
- Avoiding the skins and peel on fruit and vegetables, including the skins on baked and new potatoes
- Limiting fruit and vegetables to a maximum of five portions a day and choosing ones from the lower-fibre list (see right)
- Eating lower-fibre breakfast cereals, such as cornflakes and rice crispies

REINTRODUCING HIGHER-FIBRE FOODS

It is important to add higher-fibre foods back to the diet gradually. A sudden increase can lead to pain, wind, bloating and diarrhoea. Different people find that they can tolerate different amounts and types of fibre. Following a reintroduction programme can help to identify these more easily.

Week 1 Keep skins and peel on fruit and vegetables

Week 2 Include one portion of a higher-fibre fruit or vegetable daily (see page 17); still aim for at least 5 portions a day

Week 3 Include oat products, such as porridge and oatcakes

Week 4 Change to wholemeal bread

Week 5 Try eating wholegrain breakfast cereals

their fibre intake makes their symptoms worse. A low-fibre diet can help people whose symptoms of IBS are either diarrhoea with abdominal bloating and wind or constipation with abdominal bloating and wind.

Limiting your intake of fibre may help IBS symptoms because it will decrease the amount of bacterial fermentation that occurs in the large bowel. This will lead to less gas being produced and so reduce bloating. It will also mean that stools will be less bulky and their movement through the bowel will be slowed down.

Following a lower-fibre diet for four weeks will be long enough to know if it is going to help or not. It is a good idea to keep a record of the food and drink you take and any symptoms you experience, because it will show if there has been any improvement. If your symptoms do improve it is advisable to gradually reintroduce higher-fibre food to your diet to find a level that you can tolerate (see left).

If there has been no improvement after four weeks there is no need to remain on the diet and you should return to a normal diet.

Vegetarians and low fibre

Vegetarians who depend for their protein on pulses, lentils, nuts and seeds will have to include small portions of these foods once a day when they are on a low-fibre diet unless other sources of protein, such as milk, cheese, eggs and yogurt, are included at each meal.

Bulking agents and low-fibre diets

People who have a tendency to constipation should include a bulking agent, such as sterculia, psyllium husks, methylcellulose or linseeds, so that their constipation does not become worse. These agents can be obtained from health food shops and pharmacies. It is important to take them with plenty of fluid – say 300 ml (½ pint) – as they form a gel when eaten, which provides bulk to help stimulate a bowel motion. They should be taken every day.

Portions of fruit and vegetables

One portion of fruit is equal to 75–100 g (3–3½ oz) or 40 g (1½ oz) of dried fruit. One portion of vegetables is about 75 g (3 oz) (see right). These weights refer to the edible parts only, so skins and peel of fresh produce that are not normally eaten and the juice or water of tinned foods are not included.

Highs and lows of fruit and vegetables

The fibre content of the fruit and vegetables listed below is based on one standard portion. Fruits and vegetables that are not included in the tables have a moderate fibre intake. These can be included in the daily diet, but keep them to one portion a day.

Higher-fibre fruit and vegetables Aduki beans, apricots (dried), baked beans, baked potato with skin, blackcurrants, black eye beans, cabbage, cranberries, figs (dried), French beans, gooseberries, haricot beans, kidney beans and peas.

Lower-fibre fruit and vegetables Apple (peeled), apricots, courgettes, cucumber, grapefruit, grapes, leeks, lettuce, melon, mushrooms, nectarine (peeled), onions, peaches (peeled), peppers, radishes, tomatoes and spring onions.

GUIDE FOR ONE PORTION OF FRUIT

2 small fruits, such as fresh apricots

1 medium fruit, such as apples

1 slice of large fruit, such as melon

1 tablespoon dried fruit, such as raisins

2–3 larger dried fruits, such as dates

GUIDE FOR ONE PORTION OF VEGETABLES

3 large tablespoons cooked vegetables

Small bowl of salad

3 tablespoons beans or pulses

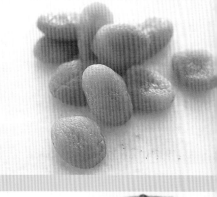

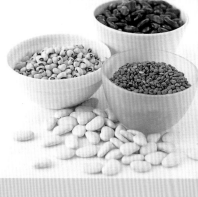

food intolerance or allergy?

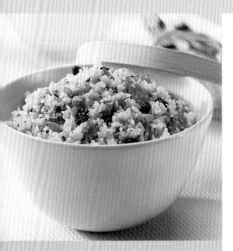

The terms food intolerance and allergy mean different things to different people. Just to confuse things even further there is also something known as food sensitivity. It is important to understand the differences between each of them.

Food allergy

An allergic response to food occurs when the body's immune system identifies a particular food as harmful to it. In response, the body produces antibodies, which can be measured by blood tests or skin prick tests. Only a small amount of the food needs to be eaten to lead to an allergic reaction. Eating the food and the appearance of symptoms can be almost immediate, but there are some conditions, such as coeliac disease (see page 24), where an allergy to a food occurs much more slowly.

'It is thought that 1–2 per cent of the general population have a food allergy, and the percentage is higher among children.'

Food intolerance

Food intolerance does not affect the immune system, and in general the symptoms take longer to occur after eating a particular food. Often, large amounts of a food have to be eaten to trigger a response. The symptoms can be similar to those of a true food allergy – rashes, diarrhoea and vomiting, for example – and for some people symptoms can be quite severe.

Testing and food intolerance

The tests used to show food allergy, such as blood tests and skin prick tests, cannot be used to identify food intolerance as it is not the result of changes in the immune system.

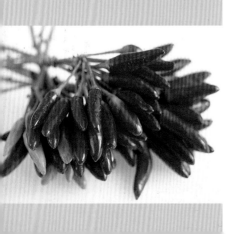

There is a wide range of tests that claim to identify food intolerance, such as hair testing, pulse testing and measuring muscle weakness. Many of these tests have not been validated and can lead to people following restricted diets for long periods, often unnecessarily. The most reliable way of determining food intolerance is to withdraw a food from the diet and see if there is an improvement in symptoms.

Causes of food intolerance

There are several different causes of food intolerance as listed below.

Digestive enzymes Some people are sensitive to particular foods because they lack the right substances in the gut, called enzymes, to digest them. An example of this would be the lack of the digestive enzyme lactase, that is needed to break down the milk sugar lactose (see page 21).

Vasoactive amines These naturally occurring substances cause the blood vessels to narrow, which can lead to headaches, nausea and giddiness. Foods rich in vasoactive amines include cheese, yeast extract, chocolate, red wine and fermented foods.

Monosodium glutamate (MSG) This flavour enhancer is found in Chinese cooking and many processed foods. Large amounts of MSG can give headaches, flushing, abdominal discomfort, chest pain and palpitations.

Irritants Some hot spices irritate the lining of the gut.

Gut bacteria There is growing evidence that the bacteria in our guts play a role in our health (see pages 36–7). Research suggests that the type of bacteria present in the large bowel may be linked with food intolerance.

SOME SYMPTOMS OF ALLERGY

- Swelling in the mouth and throat
- Runny nose (rhinitis)
- Watering eyes
- Breathing difficulties
- Skin rashes
- Small, itchy, red 'nettle rash' (urticaria)
- Diarrhoea
- Nausea and vomiting

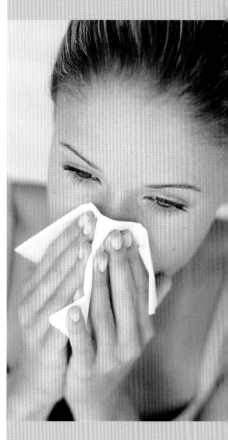

milk and dairy products

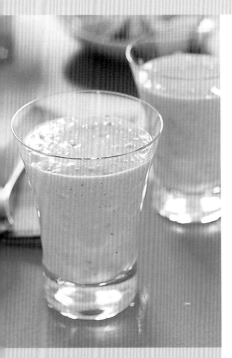

Milk is one of the most common foods linked to IBS. Research has found about 40 per cent of IBS patients following an exclusion diet identified milk as the food that upset them. It is not clear why this is the case, but some people may have an intolerance to lactose (see page 21), which is the sugar found in milk.

Lactose

Lactose is made up of two sugars, glucose and galactose, and is broken down in the small intestine by an enzyme called lactase.

As infants we produce large amounts of lactase because milk is our main food. As we get older the production of lactase decreases. If there is not enough lactase to completely break down the lactose in the small intestine, it reaches the large intestine intact, where the gut bacteria ferment it. This can give rise to symptoms of diarrhoea, bloating, pain and wind.

'Lactase production is affected by a number of factors, including ethnicity, heredity and previous illness.'

Ethnic groups

People of Asian, African and Mediterranean descent often have quite low lactase production, with 40–100 per cent of the population affected. People from Scandinavia and northern Europe retain the ability to produce lactase, and the number of people with lactase deficiency in these areas is less, at around 5 per cent.

Gastroenteritis

A bout of gastroenteritis can cause temporary damage to the lining of the small intestine and so upset the production of lactase. Some people find dairy products upset them after they have had a stomach upset.

lactose intolerance

The symptoms of lactose intolerance are very similar to those of IBS, and the number of people reported to have lactose intolerance and IBS ranges from 6 per cent to 24 per cent of the population. Research has shown that not everyone with a positive lactose breath test (see below) will improve on a low-lactose diet.

Many people with lactose intolerance can manage some lactose, sometimes as much as 250 ml (8 fl oz) milk a day, in their diet with no ill effects. A trial of a low-lactose diet for a couple of weeks may help people who include more than 300 ml (½ pint) of milk in their daily diet or if IBS symptoms started after a gut infection. In general, a milk-free diet gives better results than just excluding lactose.

Hard cheeses, such as Cheddar, and butter have only a trace of lactose and can be included in a low-lactose diet.

Testing for lactose intolerance

There are several tests available to determine lactose intolerance, but the one most often used is called a lactose hydrogen breath test. A drink containing a known amount of lactose is taken after an overnight fast. Breath samples are collected before the patient takes the drink and then every 30 minutes afterwards for two hours. If the lactose is not digested it will be fermented by the gut bacteria, which then produce hydrogen. The hydrogen enters the bloodstream and is eventually released from the lungs in the breath. A rise in hydrogen levels indicates lactose malabsorption.

MAIN SOURCES OF LACTOSE

- Milk (from a cow, goat or sheep) and foods made with milk, such as custard, white sauce, milk puddings, yogurts, ice cream and chocolates
- Lactose as a sweetener in foods and medications

a milk-free diet

DIETARY SOURCES OF MILK

- Butter and margarine
- Cakes, biscuits and baked products
- Cheese
- Chocolate
- Cream
- Crisps and savoury snacks
- Ice cream, milk puddings and desserts
- Pre-prepared meals and other convenience foods
- Vending machine drinks – hot chocolate, malted drinks and milk shakes
- Yogurt and fromage frais

ALTERNATIVES TO MILK

- Cocoa, soya milk shakes, tea, coffee, fruit and herbal teas, fruit juices and cordials
- Milk-free cakes and biscuits
- Milk-free margarine
- Plain nuts
- Ready-salted crisps
- Rice milk (calcium enriched)
- Soya cheese and soya cream
- Soya milk
- Soya yogurts, soya desserts and soya ice cream

Milk, whether from cows, sheep or goats, is found in a wide range of foods – and often where you would least expect to find it. It is important to check food labels carefully to make sure that your food is milk free. This can be difficult because of the number of different words, all meaning milk, that can be used: milk proteins (casein, caesinates, lactalbumin and whey), milk sugar (lactose) and milk fat (buttermilk). You should also keep an eye out for skimmed milk powder and milk solids.

Trial milk-free diet period

A trial of a strict milk-free diet for two or three weeks can help improve the symptoms of IBS, and keeping a food and symptoms diary (see page 31) is a helpful way of recording any changes in your symptoms. If there is no improvement after this time you should reintroduce milk to your diet.

Reintroduction of milk

If there is an improvement in the symptoms of IBS a gradual reintroduction of milk is recommended, starting with low-lactose dairy products, such as cheese or butter, and then moving on to milk itself, cream and yogurt.

It is important to test one new food at a time and to have that food on two occasions during the day. Test the food for three or four days to allow enough time for any possible reaction to occur. If the symptoms return with the inclusion of milk it does not mean you will always have to avoid it. Many people find they can include small amounts of milk on an occasional basis with no problems. It is important to re-test foods after a couple of months as an intolerance to milk can be temporary and you might find you can manage it again.

Calcium intake

Milk and milk products are excellent sources of calcium, so it is essential to include alternative sources of calcium in the diet as well. This can be done by choosing other good dietary sources of calcium (see right). Calcium-enriched soya milk or rice milk are a good choice as they contain similar amounts of calcium to cow's milk. Aim to include two to three calcium-rich foods a day. Alternatively take a calcium supplement.

GOOD SOURCES OF CALCIUM

+ Baked beans

+ Breakfast cereals (some)

+ Broccoli, spring greens, watercress and okra

+ Calcium-enriched soya and rice milks

+ Calcium-enriched soya cheese and soya yogurt

+ Sesame seeds and sesame paste (tahini)

+ Tinned sardines and pilchards (include the bones)

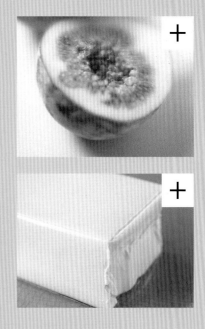

Meal plan for a milk-free diet *

Breakfast
■ Cereal with calcium-enriched soya milk with a tablespoon of dried fruit ■ Small glass of fruit juice

Lunch
■ Sandwich with milk-free margarine filled with meat or chicken or fish ■ Small mixed salad ■ Fruit or soya yogurt

Evening meal
■ Meat or chicken or fish or tofu ■ Vegetables or salad ■ Pasta, potatoes or rice ■ Fruit salad with soya ice cream

Snacks
■ Fruit ■ Milk-free bun or biscuit ■ Plain nuts ■ Ready-salted crisps (occasionally)

* Remember to drink 8–10 cups of fluid every day.

wheat

DIETARY SOURCES OF WHEAT

- Batter, such as pancakes and Yorkshire pudding
- Bread, including pitta, baguettes, rolls, muffins, crumpets and bagels
- Breadcrumbs
- Breakfast cereals (many)
- Cakes, biscuits and some confectionery
- Crackers and crispbreads
- Pasta and noodles
- Pastry

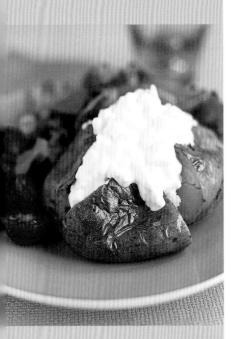

Wheat is another common food intolerance, and it has been identified by as many as 60 per cent of people with IBS who have followed an exclusion diet. It is important not to confuse a wheat-free diet with a gluten-free diet.

Gluten versus wheat

Gluten is the name given to the protein found in wheat, rye and barley. Oats contain a protein that is similar to gluten, and should initially be avoided if following a gluten-free diet. There is, however, some debate about whether complete avoidance of oats is necessary for everyone who needs a gluten-free diet. It is important to note that gluten-free foods are not always totally wheat-free as they often contain wheat starch. This makes them unsuitable for someone following a wheat-free diet.

Coeliac disease

Coeliac disease is caused by an allergy to gluten, which damages the lining of the small intestine. This can give rise to a range of symptoms, such as diarrhoea, abdominal distension, pain, anaemia, weight loss, fatigue and recurrent mouth ulcers. Treatment is purely dietary through the long-term use of a gluten-free diet.

The symptoms of coeliac disease and IBS are very similar, and it is important that coeliac disease is ruled out before a diagnosis of IBS is given. While sensitive blood tests can indicate gluten sensitivity, they are not 100 per cent accurate. The most reliable test is for a small piece of the lining of the small intestine to be removed by a doctor and looked at for signs of damage. Don't exclude gluten from the diet before these tests are carried out as this could give a negative result.

A wheat-free diet

A trial of a strict wheat-free diet can be helpful in IBS, especially if symptoms include abdominal bloating, diarrhoea and wind. Food labels can be confusing, and words that also mean 'wheat' include wheat starch, bran, wholemeal flour, flour, couscous, bulgar wheat, durum, semolina, spelt and triticum.

Avoiding wheat for two or three weeks is an adequate length of time to see an improvement. Keeping a food and symptoms diary during this time will help confirm any changes (see page 31).

If there is no change in your symptoms it is unlikely that wheat is a problem, and it should be reintroduced to your diet. If there is an improvement you should reintroduce wheat to see if it causes problems again. Eat wheat twice during the day. Some people may experience symptoms within a day, but it can take up to a week for wheat to cause a reaction.

High-fibre wheat foods can cause abdominal bloating and wind, so try white bread and white pasta for three or four days before adding wholemeal varieties.

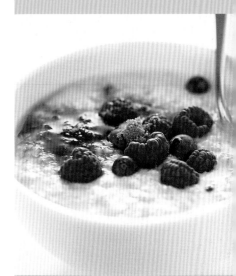

ALTERNATIVES TO WHEAT

The following list is not exhaustive, and you should always check the labels.

- Buckwheat pasta, corn pasta and rice noodles
- Corn crackers
- Oatcakes
- Rice cakes
- Rye bread (100 per cent rye flour)
- Rye crispbreads
- Wheat-free cakes and biscuits
- Porridge, some muesli, cornflakes and rice crispies

Meal plan for a wheat-free diet *

Breakfast
- Porridge ■ Fruit smoothie

Lunch
- Baked potato with filling and salad ■ Yogurt or fruit

Evening meal
- Meat or chicken or fish ■ Vegetables or salad ■ Potatoes or rice or wheat-free pasta ■ Sorbet or fruit

Snacks
- Rice cakes ■ Oatcakes ■ Plain nuts ■ Fruit

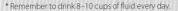

* Remember to drink 8–10 cups of fluid every day.

exclusion diets

FOODS TO AVOID ON AN EXCLUSION DIET

- Beef, processed meats, pies and pâtés
- Chocolate
- Citrus fruit and their juices and cordials
- Coffee, tea, cocoa, fizzy drinks and alcohol
- Eggs
- Fish in batter or breadcrumbs
- Milk (cow, goat or sheep) products including yogurt, cheese and ice cream
- Nuts
- Potatoes, onions, sweetcorn and vegetables tinned in sauce
- Wheat, corn, rye, barley and oats and all products made with them
- Yeast and yeast extract

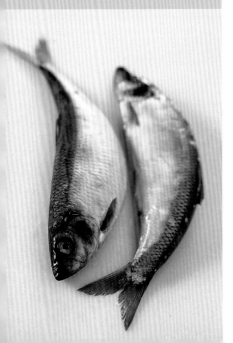

There is a group of people with IBS who find that they are intolerant of several different foods. These tend to be people who experience symptoms, such as loose or frequent bowel motions, abdominal bloating, wind and pain, several times a week or even every day. Food intolerance is more likely in those people whose symptoms started after a severe bout of gastroenteritis or after having prolonged courses of antibiotics.

Adopting an exclusion diet

An exclusion diet excludes all the most commonly reported food intolerances in one go. It is a very restricted diet and should be followed with caution and preferably with the support of an experienced dietician.

Typically, the basic diet is followed for two weeks, and it is essential that a food and symptoms diary is kept throughout this time (see page 31) to record if there has been any improvement over the exclusion period. If there is no change in symptoms over this time the diet should be stopped and a normal diet resumed. If there is an improvement then the excluded foods should be reintroduced back to the diet one at a time.

Are you prepared?

Although an exclusion diet can be helpful in identifying food intolerance it should not be undertaken lightly, as it can make life difficult.

Eating out can be tricky, especially during the initial two-week period. Don't be embarrassed to ask about ingredients used or if a meal can be adapted for you.

There are few ready-prepared foods available that are suitable for the basic diet, so be prepared to make meals from scratch – making them in bulk will save you time. Shopping may also take longer because you have to check food labels to make sure the product is free from all foods excluded on the basic diet.

Ensure your diet is nutritionally balanced by following healthy eating guidelines (pages 11–12) and by including a variety of foods on a daily basis. Take the opportunity to try new or unfamiliar foods and recipes.

Finding suitable snacks or eating away from home can be inconvenient or difficult, so you have to be organized and take suitable food with you.

FOODS ALLOWED ON AN EXCLUSION DIET

- All other meat, chicken and game
- All other fruit, their juices and cordials
- All other vegetables, fresh, frozen and canned
- Dairy-free margarine
- Fruit and herbal teas
- Rice milk (calcium-enriched)
- Rice, millet, quinoa and buckwheat
- Seeds
- Soya milk (calcium-enriched), soya yogurts, soya ice cream and soya cheese
- Sugar, syrup and honey
- White and oily fish and shellfish

Meal plan for a basic exclusion diet *

Breakfast
- Rice cereal with sliced banana and calcium-enriched soya milk
- Glass of apple juice

Lunch
- Cold chicken or ham with salad and rice cakes with dairy-free spread ■ Soya yogurt

Evening meal
- Pork chop with apple sauce ■ Vegetables and rice ■ Mixed berries with soya ice cream

Snacks
- Fruit ■ Seeds ■ Vegetable crisps ■ Carob bar (check that it is milk-free) ■ Sesame snaps

Note The exclusion diet is not suitable during pregnancy or for women who are breastfeeding. If you are diabetic you should discuss the diet with your doctor before undertaking it.

* Remember to drink 8–10 cups of fluid every day.

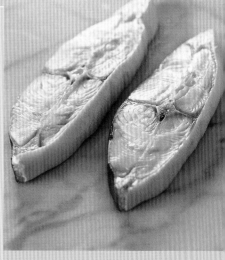

food reintroduction

'Pure foods need to be reintroduced before foods that contain them, such as yeast before wine and bread.'

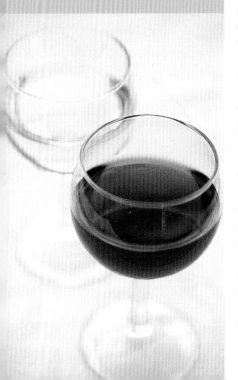

After two weeks on the exclusion diet food should be reintroduced to your diet. Take two days to test each food, as it can take 24–36 hours for a food to give a reaction. Wheat should be tested for seven days, because it can take longer for symptoms to return. If problems do occur, stop eating the food being tested and wait for symptoms to clear before trying the next food.

One food at a time

The amount of food tested is important. Having a small portion of a food once during the day may not be enough to give a reaction, so it is usually suggested that two portions of the test food are eaten. Also, don't test more than one food at a time, because this can lead to confusion and prolong the time on the exclusion diet.

Some test foods are found as ingredients in other foods, so it is important that these are tried first – for example, yeast needs to be tried before wine or bread and milk before cheese, yogurt or butter.

Once the food reintroduction phase is complete the foods that provoke symptoms should be avoided for another three to six months. After this time it is advisable to re-test these foods, because quite often people find they are able to tolerate them after they have been avoided for a long period.

It is unusual to find more than three or four foods that cause symptoms. However, sometimes many foods appear to cause problems. For this group of people an assessment by a dietician is strongly recommended to make sure that their basic diet is nutritionally adequate and to give advice on suitable alternatives to the foods that are being avoided.

Suggested order of food reintroduction

Food	Suggested amount for one portion *
Potatoes	1 large jacket potato; 2–3 egg-sized boiled potatoes; 2 serving spoons of mash (use milk-free margarine); a small portion of chips cooked in suitable oil; 2–3 egg-sized roast potatoes
Beef	75–100 g (3–3½ oz)
Yeast	3 brewer's yeast tablets a day
Cows' milk	A minimum of 300 ml (½ pint) during the day, preferably 600 ml (1 pint) a day; can be tested as whole, semi-skimmed or skimmed milk; use it in drinks or as an ingredient in dishes such as rice pudding
Rye	3–4 rye crispbreads; 1–2 slices of rye bread if yeast is tolerated (check that it is 100 per cent rye flour)
Tea	No more than 4–5 cups a day
Butter or margarine	25–50 g (1–2 oz) during the day
Corn	4 tablespoons of cornflakes; 2 tablespoons of sweetcorn or 1 corn-on-the-cob; cornflour in sauces; 2–3 corn crackers; vegetable oil can also be included
Eggs	2 during the day; egg as an ingredient in other food
White wine	A maximum of 3 glasses a day if yeast is tolerated
Citrus fruits	1 orange; ½ a grapefruit; small glass of citrus fruit juice; 2 satsumas, tangerines, mandarins or clementines; lemon juice in cooking; citrus fruit squashes
Oats	3–4 oatcakes; 3–4 tablespoons of dry oats for porridge; 1 piece of flapjack
Chocolate	3–4 teaspoons of cocoa; 3–4 teaspoons of hot chocolate powder; 50 g (2 oz) chocolate if milk tolerated
Cheese	25–40 g (1–1½ oz); cheese made with goats' or ewes' milk should be tested separately
Wheat	1–2 slices of bread (if yeast is tolerated); 5–6 tablespoons of pasta; 2 Weetabix or Shredded Wheat; 4 tablespoons bran flakes
Coffee	No more than 3–4 cups a day
Yogurt	1 small pot or 3 tablespoons; yogurt made with goats' or ewes' milk should be tested separately
Nuts	A small handful unsalted or salted nuts; choose the type you would most commonly eat
Barley	Pearl barley in a casserole; barley water squashes; 3–4 tablespoons breakfast cereal containing barley
Vinegar	In salad dressing, sauces or added to food
Fizzy drinks	No more than 3 glasses (600 ml or 1 pint) a day

* You need to have two portions a day unless otherwise stated

other diet-related triggers

SOURCES OF SORBITOL

- Fruit: plums, cherries, pears and prunes
- Diabetic products: marmalade, jam and chocolate
- Sugar-free products: chewing gum and mints

SOURCES OF FRUCTOSE

- Fruit, such as apples, bananas, cherries, grapes and pears
- Dried fruit, such as apricots, currants, figs, raisins and sultanas
- Fruit juices, such as apple, grape, grapefruit and prune

TIPS FOR CUTTING FAT INTAKE INCLUDE

- Grill, bake, steam foods rather than fry them
- Change to low-fat products
- Trim visible fat from meat and take the skin off chicken
- Avoid pastry
- Steer clear of creamy sauces and try tomato-based ones instead
- Limit your intake of crisps, savoury snacks, chocolate, biscuits and cakes to a couple of times a week

Some evidence suggests that some people with IBS are sensitive to certain sugars found within foods, such as fruit sugar (fructose) and milk sugar (lactose) and a sugar-alcohol called sorbitol. Fatty foods can also cause IBS symptoms.

Sorbitol

Sorbitol, often used as a sweetener in sugar-free and diabetic products and some medications, is also found naturally in certain fruits. An intake of 30 g (about 1 oz) a day is known to give stomach cramps, flatulence and diarrhoea, but lower intakes can cause symptoms.

Fructose

Some people with IBS complain of abdominal bloating and discomfort after being given fructose under test conditions. There is, however, no evidence that this is due to a true malabsorption of fructose, but it is thought that some IBS sufferers may have a heightened sensitivity to it. If foods rich in both fructose and sorbitol are eaten symptoms may be seen with much smaller portions of food.

Fatty foods

Rich or fatty foods are often linked with bowel problems. When fat is eaten it causes the body to release a substance called cholecystokinin (CCK) – a stimulant of colonic motility. This can cause pain, which is often mistaken for gallstones. Fatty foods can also give indigestion, abdominal discomfort and diarrhoea.

Spicy foods

Highly spiced foods have also been linked with indigestion, abdominal discomfort and diarrhoea.

the symptom-linked approach

Unfortunately, there is no one treatment for the symptoms of IBS, and everyone responds differently to different treatments. However, identifying the main symptoms allows you to follow a more structured approach in finding the most appropriate way of controlling them. The use of a food, lifestyle and symptoms diary can prove helpful in identifying any patterns between diet and symptoms, stress or a combination of factors. Women can also find it worth making a note of their menstrual cycles.

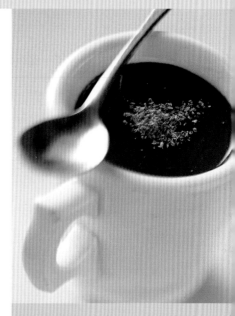

Keeping a symptoms diary

A small notebook is ideal for a symptoms diary, but some people prefer to keep it on their computer. You will need to keep the diary for a minimum of two weeks, although longer will be necessary if you experience symptoms less frequently than that or if there is a possible link to your menstrual cycle. You will need to keep a note of the information listed (see right).

Using the information

The information recorded in the diary will help you in a number of ways.

First of all, it will identify the main symptoms you are suffering and how often you are experiencing them. The diary should help you spot a link between a particular food and your symptoms, perhaps helping you identify if there is a link with fatty, spicy or rich foods, for example.

DIARY NOTES

- The time of eating, any symptoms or any other event
- A general description of the food eaten at each meal – for example, white pasta with tomato sauce rather than just 'pasta'
- The fluid taken – that is, the type of drink (including alcohol) and the amount
- A clear description of the symptoms – pain on right-hand side, loose bowel motion, hard, pellet-like motion, needed to rush to the toilet, and so on
- If you have had a particularly stressful or emotional day
- If you have taken any exercise or have been sitting down all day

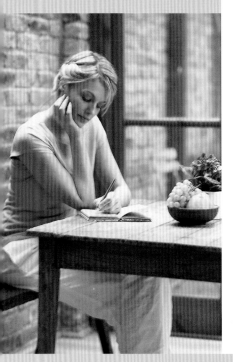

It will also reveal if you have an irregular meal pattern or if you eat differently during the week and highlight if you have a low- or high-fibre diet or if your intake of fibre alters a lot from day to day.

The diary will help you work out if you are having enough to drink and show if you are having too many fizzy drinks, caffeine or alcohol. It will also make you think about the portion sizes of your meals and how you eat your food.

Noting how you feel will enable you to see if stress or anxiety play a part, and the diary will also reveal if the amount of exercise – or lack of exercise – has any effect on your symptoms.

Once you have established which are your main symptoms, you will be in a much better position to decide on the best way of changing your diet to help you manage your IBS.

Example 'symptoms' diary

Date	Time	Food eaten	Time	Symptoms and comments
Mon 26	7.30 am	2 slices white toast with butter and jam; cup of tea		
	During morning	3 cups of coffee and 1 apple	11.00 am	busy at work, feel stressed
		missed lunch		
			2.00 pm	headache, tummy pains
	3.00 pm	2 cups of tea and a chocolate bar		
	7.00 pm	chicken with new potatoes, peas and broccoli; yogurt; glass of red wine		
	8.00 pm	glass of red wine		
	9.00 pm	cup of tea and a biscuit		

symptom-linked groups

Although the symptoms of IBS vary from person to person, there are three main groups of symptoms into which most people fit. The three groups are: mostly diarrhoea; episodes of diarrhoea then constipation (alternating bowel habit); and mostly constipation. There may also be other symptoms present, such as abdominal pain or discomfort, abdominal bloating, flatulence, urgency to open the bowels, indigestion or acid reflux, tiredness and headaches.

Before making any radical changes to your diet it is important that you are following a healthy, balanced diet with an adequate fluid intake (see pages 11–13). Don't forget the importance of regular meals, taking time over eating and moderating your portion sizes. Quite often symptoms improve just by making these simple changes. It is also important to allow time for your body to get used to any dietary changes. Improvements are unlikely to happen overnight, and it may take several weeks to notice a change. Continuing with a food and symptoms diary will be helpful because it will highlight if there has been any improvement in symptoms or not.

Mostly diarrhoea

If you are in this group your main symptom is loose, frequent bowel motions at least once a week. Other symptoms may include abdominal bloating, abdominal discomfort or pain, flatulence (wind) and urgency to open the bowels.

DIETARY CHANGES FOR ALL SYMPTOM GROUPS

No matter which symptom group you are in, before you make any major changes to your diet it is important to:

- Follow a healthy, balanced diet
- Have an adequate fluid intake (8–10 cups of fluid a day)
- Have a regular meal pattern
- Keep a food and symptoms diary
- Check excessive intakes of caffeine, alcohol, spicy foods, fatty foods, fructose and sorbitol

MAINLY DIARRHOEA GROUP

- Low-fibre diet
- Single-food exclusion
- Exclusion diet

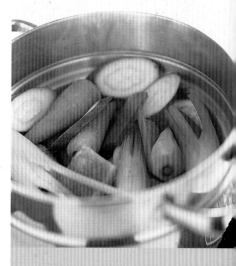

ALTERNATING DIARRHOEA AND CONSTIPATION GROUP

Alternating bowel habit without wind and bloating

- High-fibre diet with the addition of a bulking agent if needed
- Single-food exclusion
- Exclusion diet

Alternating bowel habit with wind and bloating

- Low-fibre diet with bulking agent if needed
- Single-food exclusion
- Exclusion diet

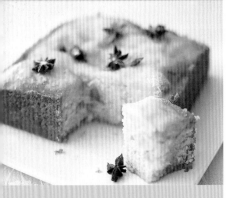

The first dietary change to make is to follow a lower-fibre diet (see pages 15–17) for three or four weeks. The addition of a fibre supplement or a bulking agent (see pages 15–17) may be necessary to prevent constipation. If there is no improvement after four weeks it is important to return to a normal diet.

If a low-fibre diet is unsuccessful it might be that a particular food is causing your symptoms. This is more likely if IBS started after gastroenteritis or a stomach upset, or after a long course of antibiotics, and diarrhoea is occurring several times a week. Reviewing your symptoms diary may give you an indication of which food is responsible. The most common intolerances are milk and wheat, and a trial of a milk-free or a wheat-free diet – or both – can prove helpful (see pages 22–5). If your symptoms occur every day a full exclusion diet (see pages 26–7) might be the best approach.

Alternating diarrhoea and constipation

If you are in this group your main symptom is loose or frequent bowel motions, followed by several days or weeks of a normal regular bowel habit. You will then find your bowel motions become less frequent and the motions become hard and pellet-like and more difficult to pass. Other symptoms may include abdominal bloating and flatulence (wind).

If you switch from diarrhoea to constipation with no abdominal bloating and wind, try to gradually increase your fibre intake. At the same time make sure that you have an adequate fluid intake (see page 13).

If you find increasing your dietary fibre difficult the use of a fibre substitute or bulking agent (see pages 15–17) can be helpful. It is important to follow a high-fibre diet for several weeks and to keep a food and symptoms diary to monitor any change in symptoms. If increasing fibre intake is not helpful after about four weeks try an exclusion diet (see pages 26–7).

For those people who have an alternating bowel habit accompanied by abdominal bloating and wind a lower-fibre diet is often helpful (see pages 15–17). Again, a good fluid intake is essential. To prevent constipation becoming worse a bulking agent will help regulate bowel motions until higher-fibre foods are reintroduced to the diet (see pages 16–17). If there is no improvement after four weeks it is possible that there is a food intolerance and trying a single-food exclusion or a full exclusion diet can prove helpful.

Mostly constipation

The main symptom of people in this group is an infrequent bowel motion that can be painful to pass. Other symptoms may include abdominal bloating, abdominal pain and flatulence (wind).

One person may say they are constipated if they don't pass a bowel motion every day, whereas another may say they are constipated if they open their bowels once a week. Generally, it is described as a bowel motion less than twice a week with the passage of hard, pellet-like or thin, flat, ribbon-like motions. Straining to pass a stool is often experienced together with abdominal pain.

Some people have sluggish bowels and need regular laxatives to stimulate a bowel motion. Such people should be under the supervision of a doctor. The continued use of laxatives is not recommended as the body can become dependent on them, and increased amounts are needed to have the same effect.

Where constipation without bloating and wind is the main symptom it is important to have an adequate fibre and fluid intake (see pages 13 and 15).

If constipation is the main symptom with abdominal bloating and wind, a lower-fibre diet plus a daily bulking agent, such as psyllium husks or linseeds (see pages 15–17), can help to improve symptoms.

MAINLY CONSTIPATION

Constipation without bloating and wind

- High-fibre diet

Constipation with bloating and wind

- Low-fibre diet with bulking agent if needed

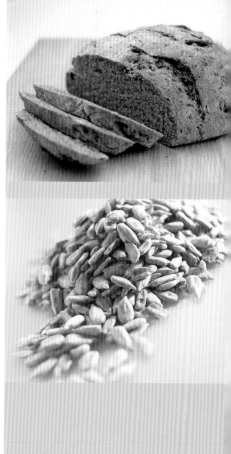

probiotics and prebiotics

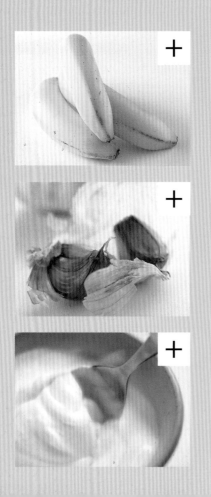

Everyone has billions of bacteria living in their large bowel. There are hundreds of different types of bacteria that in general live in a balance together. Certain types of bacteria – 'good' or 'friendly' bacteria – are beneficial to the body. They also help to keep harmful bacteria under control.

Upsetting the balance

When the balance of good and bad bacteria is altered it can lead to problems such as diarrhoea, bloating, wind, constipation, discomfort and generally feeling below par. This balance can be altered if you take antibiotics, or after a bout of food poisoning or 'traveller's' diarrhoea. It can also be affected by a diet that contains little fruit and vegetables but is high in fat and alcohol.

What is a probiotic?

Probiotic is the name given to live 'good' bacteria. These can be taken as a supplement or added to food items. They are available in a wide range of products, including yogurts and yogurt drinks, and they are added to fruit juices and are available in capsule form. There is a lot of interest in the use of probiotics, and there is growing evidence that they:

- ☐ Boost the immune system
- ☐ Increase resistance to infection
- ☐ Help in the prevention and treatment of diarrhoea resulting from bacterial infection
- ☐ Help to prevent diarrhoea resulting from antibiotic therapy
- ☐ Improve movement of the bowel
- ☐ May improve mild inflammation of the bowel

At present there are no guidelines on the amount of probiotic that should be taken. More research is needed to work out how much and which types of bacteria are needed and the best way that they can reach the large intestine unharmed.

What is a prebiotic?

A prebiotic is a food substance that specifically promotes the growth of good bacteria in the bowel. These foods need to resist being digested in the small intestine so that they arrive relatively unchanged in the large bowel. The most commonly used ones are fructo-oligosaccharides (FOS) and inulin. Many probiotic supplements or foods now have prebiotics added to them as well.

Who needs probiotics and prebiotics?

Research shows that probiotics are a promising therapy for a wide range of health problems, including IBS, lactose intolerance and gastrointestinal infections. Probiotics may also lower cholesterol levels and reduce the risk of cancer.

A trial of a probiotic may be worth undertaking if you have recently had an upset stomach or have started a course of antibiotics that has triggered your IBS. In general, they are safe to take for most people of all ages. However, if your immune system is not working properly or if you are taking drugs that affect your immune system – some cancer treatments, for example – you should avoid probiotics.

Capsules that have a combination of probiotics and a prebiotic, which have a special coating that resists digestion in the stomach, are a good choice. Yogurts and yogurt drinks must be kept chilled, and the longer they are kept the more likely it is that the bacteria will die. These yogurts are not suitable for people with a milk intolerance.

A GOOD PROBIOTIC WILL NEED TO:

- Contain bacteria that can reach the large intestine without being damaged
- Contain large numbers of bacteria
- Be taken on a daily basis
- Have more than one type of bacteria, such as *Acidophillus* and *Bifidobacteria* bacteria

some questions answered

Is there any drug treatment for IBS?
▶

There are various types of medication available to help control the symptoms of IBS; however, they do not cure the problem. These include:

- ☐ Anti-spasmodics to decrease muscular spasm in the gut
- ☐ Laxatives to treat constipation
- ☐ Medications to slow down the movement of the gut to control diarrhoea
- ☐ Pain relief to control abdominal pain and discomfort
- ☐ Tranquillizers, which appear to help improve IBS symptoms

Most medications have unwanted side-effects, and not all medications are suitable for all people. You should discuss possible drug treatments with your doctor or pharmacist to ensure it is right for you.

Will I always have IBS?
▶

Most people find that their IBS symptoms come and go and that the symptoms become less severe with time. Symptoms are often triggered by a period of illness, stress or upheaval.

It is important not to link all bowel symptoms with IBS. If you have a change in your symptoms, have rectal bleeding or blood in your stools, experience sudden unexplained weight loss or a change to your normal bowel habit, you should have this checked by your doctor. These can be signs of more serious problems.

What is candida and is there a link with IBS?
▶

Candida albicans is a yeast-like fungus, which occurs naturally in the body. If the normal levels of bacteria in the gut are altered – which can happen after an infection or taking antibiotics – the candida can grow rapidly, resulting in thrush. Some people think this can lead to intolerance of yeast and yeast products and that avoiding them and sugary foods, which stimulate their growth, will improve symptoms of abdominal bloating, wind and pain. There is, however, currently inadequate evidence to support the use of anti-candida diets in the management of IBS.

Do I need to take any vitamin or mineral supplements?
▶

If you follow a balanced diet it is unlikely that you will require any vitamin and mineral supplements. However, there are some instances when a particular vitamin or mineral may be needed, including:

- ☐ Calcium for people following a milk-free diet
- ☐ Multivitamin and mineral for those on an exclusion diet
- ☐ Iron, folic acid or vitamin B12 for those who are anaemic
- ☐ Evening primrose oil for those whose IBS symptoms are linked with their menstrual cycle

Multivitamin and mineral tablets often contain lactose (milk sugar), wheat, corn (maize), yeast and other food items, so it is important that you choose a make that is suitable for your particular food intolerance.

Large doses of single vitamins and minerals are not recommended. Keep to ones that supply no more than the Recommended Daily Intake (RDI) unless otherwise advised by a doctor or dietician. Excessive intake of certain vitamins and minerals can be dangerous or lead to unpleasant side-effects. For example, vitamin C in levels over 1 g can result in abdominal discomfort and diarrhoea.

Does stress affect IBS?
▶

Yes, some people find that stressful situations can lead to diarrhoea and abdominal pain. It can also lead to anxiety and a faster, shallow breathing pattern. Continued stress can give disturbed sleep and eating patterns, which in turn make IBS symptoms worse.

Finding a way to tackle stress, such as learning relaxation techniques and yoga, will help to decrease stress. Thirty minutes of moderate exercise five days a week is also helpful as exercise stimulates the body to produce feel-good substances called endorphins.

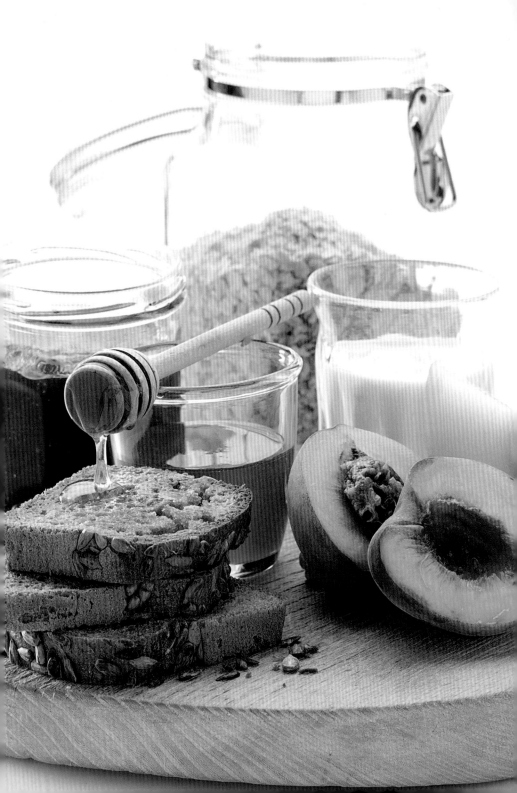

breakfasts

Nutrition
Gluten free, wheat free
Kcals 298
Fat 13 g
Saturated fat 6 g
Sodium 320 mg
Fibre 4 g

Preparation time
15 minutes
Cooking time
8–10 minutes
Serves
4

NUTRITIONAL TIP
Use stewed sliced peaches, nectarines or apples to lower the fibre content.

american cinnamon pancakes

Avoiding wheat and foods that contain gluten can limit breakfasts somewhat. Topped with natural yogurt, mixed berries and a drizzle of maple syrup, these thick, griddle-style pancakes are lovely for a relaxed weekend breakfast.

250 g (8 oz) frozen fruits of the forest

2 tablespoons water

40 g (1½ oz) fine cornmeal (masa harina)

40 g (1½ oz) tapioca flour

½ teaspoon ground cinnamon

1 teaspoon bicarbonate of soda

200 ml (7 fl oz) low-fat yogurt

1 egg

1 tablespoon sunflower oil

Greek yogurt, to serve

maple syrup or clear honey, to serve

1 Put the frozen fruit into a small saucepan with the measured water, cover and simmer for 4–5 minutes until hot.

2 Put the flours, cinnamon and bicarbonate of soda into a small bowl and stir together. Add the low-fat yogurt and egg and whisk together briefly until just mixed and smooth.

3 Lightly oil and heat a large, nonstick frying pan or griddle. Drop 6 large spoonfuls of the batter into the pan, spacing them well apart, and cook for about 2 minutes until the top has bubbled and the underside is browned. Turn over and cook the other side in the same way.

4 Remove the pancakes from the pan, keep hot on a plate, add more oil if necessary and make 6 more pancakes in the same way. Serve 3 pancakes per portion, each topped with spoonfuls of fruit, some yogurt and a drizzle of maple syrup or honey.

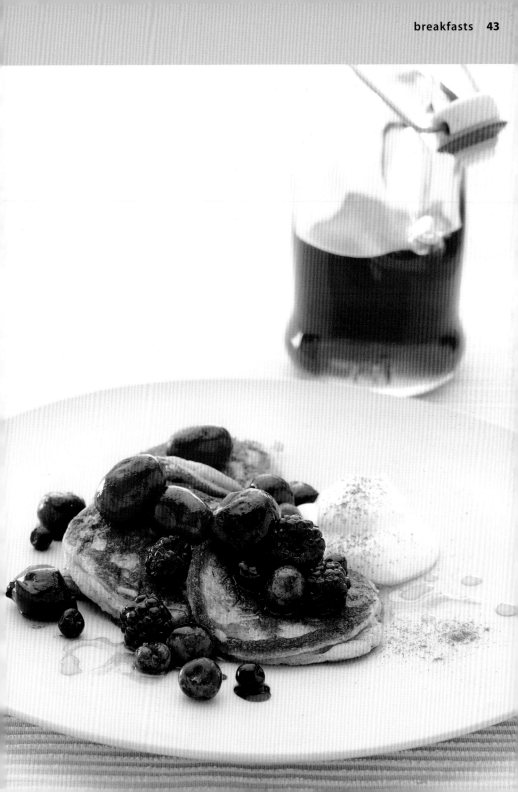

Nutrition
Wheat free, gluten free, high fibre
Kcals 343
Fat 8 g
Saturated fat 4 g
Sodium 127 mg
Fibre 5 g

Preparation time
5 minutes
Cooking time
4–5 minutes
Serves
4

NUTRITIONAL TIP
Use unsweetened soya milk instead of
dairy milk if you prefer. If you use soya
yogurt rather than Greek yogurt this dish
will be suitable for an exclusion diet.

mixed grain porridge

Quick and easy to make, this blend of buckwheat, quinoa and millet flakes gives a
finished porridge that has a slightly smoother texture than one made from rolled oats.

50 g (2 oz) buckwheat flakes

50 g (2 oz) quinoa flakes

50 g (2 oz) millet flakes

**600 ml (1 pint) semi-skimmed
milk**

300 ml (½ pint) water

2 bananas

4 tablespoons Greek yogurt

**clear honey or maple syrup,
to serve**

**sprinkling of ground
cinnamon, to serve**

1 Put the grain flakes, milk and water into a saucepan and
bring to the boil, reduce the heat and cook for 4–5 minutes,
stirring until thickened.

2 Mash one of the bananas and slice the other. Stir the
mashed banana into the porridge, spoon into bowls and
top with spoonfuls of yogurt, the sliced banana, a drizzle of
honey or maple syrup and a sprinkling of cinnamon.

Nutrition

Dairy free

Kcals 229

Fat 6 g

Saturated fat 1 g

Sodium 120 mg

Fibre 3 g

Preparation time

15 minutes

Cooking time

15–20 minutes

Makes

10 muffins

NUTRITIONAL TIP

Mixing wholemeal and white flour is a good way to get the best of both worlds, but all wholemeal or all white flour will work just as well – the fibre content either increases or reduces.

carrot and cinnamon muffins

Serve these muffins straight from the oven either plain or spread with a little low-fat soft cheese and apricot jam for a special weekend breakfast treat. Any leftovers can be packed into lunchboxes or frozen for another day.

125 g (4 oz) self-raising wholemeal flour

100 g (3½ oz) self-raising white flour

100 g (3½ oz) soft dark muscovado sugar

1 teaspoon ground cinnamon

25 g (1 oz) ready-chopped glacé ginger or stem ginger, drained and chopped

200 g (7 oz) carrots, grated

50 g (2 oz) raisins or sultanas

2 eggs

4 tablespoons sunflower oil

grated rind of 1 orange

6 tablespoons orange juice

3 tablespoons golden syrup

2 tablespoons barley flakes or porridge oats (optional)

1 Put the flours, sugar, cinnamon, ginger, carrots and raisins or sultanas into a mixing bowl.

2 Mix together the eggs, oil, orange rind and juice and add to the dry ingredients along with the golden syrup. Fork together until just mixed.

3 Line 10 sections of a deep muffin tin with paper cases and spoon the mixture into the cases. Sprinkle with barley flakes or oats (if used) and bake in a preheated oven, 190°C (375°F), Gas Mark 5, for 15–20 minutes or until well risen and the tops are slightly cracked. Serve warm.

Nutrition

Dairy free, wheat free

Kcals 250

Fat 16 g

Saturated fat 2 g

Sodium 7 mg

Fibre 3 g

Preparation time

10 minutes

Cooking time

8–10 minutes

Serves

6

NUTRITIONAL TIP

If you have a nut allergy, omit the nuts and add extra grains instead. If you omit the barley flakes and only use porridge oats, millet and quinoa, this dish is suitable for an exclusion diet.

honeyed granola

This crunchy, caramelized breakfast cereal is packed with grains, nuts and seeds. Serve it broken into pieces with dairy, rice or soya milk or a mix of berry fruits and low-fat yogurt. Try adding a little ground cinnamon or ginger to the mixture before baking.

3 tablespoons clear honey

3 tablespoons sunflower oil

50 g (2 oz) porridge oats or barley flakes

50 g (2 oz) millet or quinoa flakes

50 g (2 oz) mixed seeds, including 2 or more of sesame, sunflower, pumpkin and linseeds

50 g (2 oz) whole hazelnuts, cashew nuts or almonds or a mixture, roughly chopped

1 Warm the honey and oil in a medium-sized saucepan. Stir in the remaining ingredients and mix well.

2 Tip the mixture into a lightly oiled deep baking sheet or roasting tin and spread it into a thin, even layer. Roast in a preheated oven, 180°C (350°F), Gas Mark 4, for 6–8 minutes.

3 Remove from the oven, stir well, moving the paler mixture from the centre to the outer edges, and cook for 2 more minutes until evenly browned. Stir well.

4 Leave to cool, then transfer to an airtight storage jar. Keep for up to 7 days.

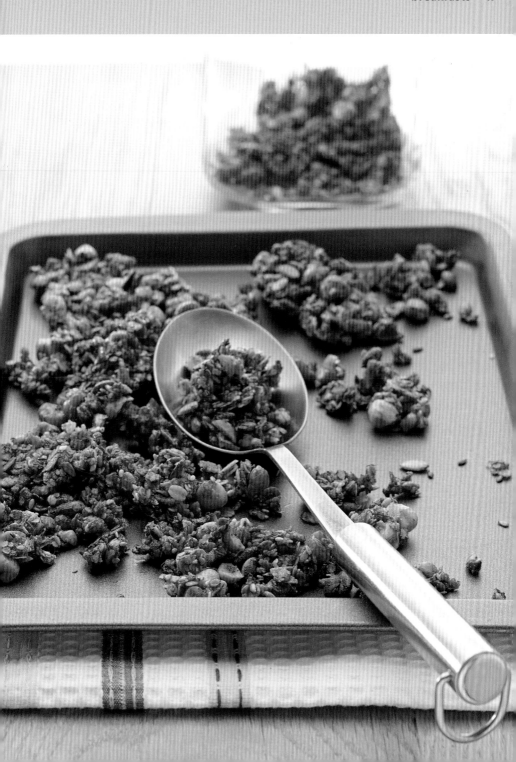

Nutrition

High fibre, milk free

Kcals 246

Fat 1 g

Saturated fat 0 g

Sodium 113 mg

Fibre 4 g

Preparation time

20 minutes, plus

soaking

Cooking time

about 1 hour 10 minutes

Makes

10 slices

NUTRITIONAL TIP

This is a good choice for a low-fat, high-fibre snack or dessert.

pineapple, date and sultana bread

This easy, yeast-free bread keeps well and is useful for those rushed mornings when you need a breakfast you can take with you. Serve thinly spread with butter or low-fat spread and have a banana or extra piece of fruit.

220 g can pineapple slices in natural juice

100 g (3½ oz) stoned dates

200 g (7 oz) sultanas

200 ml (7 fl oz) pineapple juice

100 g (3½ oz) caster sugar

150 g (5 oz) self-raising wholemeal flour

150 g (5 oz) self-raising white flour

1 egg

1 Drain the pineapple and pour the juice into a small saucepan. Finely chop the pineapple slices and roughly chop the dates. Put the pineapple, dates and sultanas into a mixing bowl.

2 Add the measured pineapple juice to the juice from the can. Bring to the boil, pour over the fruit and leave to stand for 4 hours or longer if preferred.

3 Mix the remaining ingredients into the soaked fruit. Spoon into a lightly oiled and lined 1 kg (2 lb) loaf tin and level the top. Bake in a preheated oven, 160°C, 325°F, Gas Mark 3, for about 1 hour 10 minutes (check after 1 hour) or until well risen and a skewer inserted into the centre of the loaf comes out cleanly.

4 Leave to cool in the tin, then take out and peel away the lining paper. Wrap in foil or store in an airtight container for up to 7 days. Slice and serve plain or lightly buttered.

Nutrition
Dairy free, gluten free
Kcals 227
Fat 14 g
Saturated fat 3 g
Sodium 10 mg
Fibre 2 g

Preparation time
10 minutes
Cooking time
none
Serves
2

NUTRITIONAL TIP
Use soya milk and soya yogurt to make
the drinks suitable for a milk-free diet.

minty avocado smoothie

If you are a reluctant fruit eater then one of these refreshing, vibrantly coloured,
vitamin-boosting drinks can be the perfect way to start the day.

1 ripe avocado, halved, stoned

3 stems of mint

juice of 1 lime

450 ml (¾ pint) apple juice

1 Scoop the flesh out of the avocado skin into a liquidizer or
food processor. Add the mint, lime and half the apple juice.

2 Blend until smooth and then add the remaining apple
juice and mix briefly. Pour into 2 glasses.

ALTERNATIVES
Tropical sunrise Put into a liquidizer or food processor
1 large ripe mango, stoned and peeled, 1 ripe nectarine or
peach, quartered and stoned, 300 ml (½ pint) orange juice
and 1 tablespoon chopped glacé or stem ginger. Blend until
smooth. Pour into 2 glasses.

Spiced banana Put into a liquidizer or food processor
1 large ripe banana, about 225 g (7½ oz) with skin on, thickly
sliced, ¼ teaspoon ground cinnamon, 2 teaspoons clear
honey, 125 g (4 oz) low-fat Greek yogurt and 200 ml (7 fl oz)
semi-skimmed milk. Blend until smooth. Pour into 2 glasses.

Nutrition
Wheat and gluten free, low fibre
Kcals 187
Fat 8 g
Saturated fat 4 g
Sodium 197 mg
Fibre 1 g

Preparation time
15 minutes
Cooking time
30 minutes
Makes
10 slices

NUTRITIONAL TIP
If you don't need to avoid wheat or gluten, use white flour instead for a low-fibre treat.

quick cheese bread

Try this savoury bread warm from the oven with sliced ham and tomatoes or toasted and cut into fingers with a softly boiled egg for a tasty gluten-free breakfast. If you don't have any mustard powder, mix 2 teaspoons Dijon mustard into the milk, but check that it is gluten free.

250 g (8 oz) gluten- and wheat-free white bread flour with natural gum

¼ teaspoon salt

2½ teaspoons gluten-free baking powder

1 teaspoon gluten-free mustard powder

100 g (3½ oz) mature Cheddar cheese, grated

300 ml (½ pint) semi-skimmed milk

2 eggs

50 g (2 oz) reduced-fat spread, melted

1 tablespoon sesame seeds (optional)

1 Put all the dry ingredients into a mixing bowl and add the cheese. Put the milk, eggs and melted spread into a large jug and fork together. Gradually mix into the dry ingredients and then stir until smooth.

2 Pour the mixture into a lightly oiled 1 kg (2 lb) loaf tin, level the surface and sprinkle with the sesame seeds (if used). Bake in a preheated oven, 180°C (350°F), Gas Mark 4, for about 30 minutes or until well risen and a skewer comes out cleanly when inserted into the centre.

3 Leave to cool for 10 minutes, then loosen the edge of the bread and turn it out. Serve warm, cold or toasted and spread with a little reduced-fat spread.

Nutrition

Wheat and gluten free, low fibre

Kcals 187

Fat 8 g

Saturated fat 4 g

Sodium 197 mg

Fibre 1 g

Preparation time

15 minutes

Cooking time

about 15 minutes

Serves

4

✚ **NUTRITIONAL TIP**

If you are serving this dish to a vegetarian, omit the bacon and Worcestershire sauce, drizzling the mushrooms with a little balsamic vinegar instead. If you are on a gluten-free diet, you might want to omit the Worcestershire sauce, just in case.

brunch special

All the flavour of a fry-up but without the calories or fat, not to mention the indigestion afterwards. Choose deep, well-rounded mushrooms so that there is a good cavity to drop the egg into. If the mushrooms are quite flat put a large biscuit cutter over the top of the mushroom or put the mushroom into an oiled individual tart tin so that the cutter or tin holds the egg in place.

4 deep field mushrooms, each a little over 75 g (3 oz)

25 g (1 oz) reduced-fat spread

8 rashers of smoked back bacon, 250 g (8 oz) in total

4 tomatoes, halved

4 teaspoons Worcestershire sauce

4 eggs

salt and pepper

chopped chives, to garnish

granary toast (or white toast for a low-fibre diet), to serve

1 Remove the stems from the mushrooms and place the tops on a baking sheet, the black gills uppermost. Add a knob of spread to each and season. Lay the bacon over the top and arrange the tomatoes around the mushrooms.

2 Bake in a preheated oven, 200°C (400°F), Gas Mark 6, for 10 minutes, then lift the bacon off the mushrooms and put it onto the baking sheet. Drizzle the Worcestershire sauce into each mushroom and break an egg in the centre of each. Season the eggs, then return the baking sheet to the oven.

3 Bake for 4–5 minutes or until the eggs are just set and the bacon is cooked. Transfer to serving plates and sprinkle with chopped chives. Serve with granary toast.

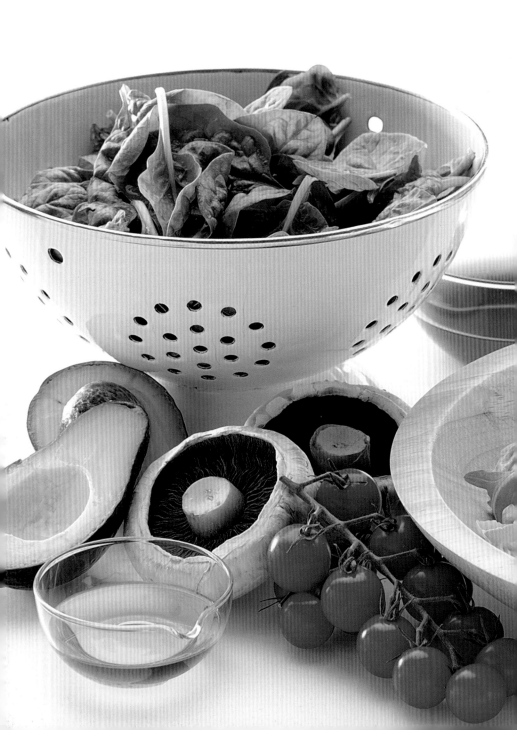

light
bites

Nutrition

Wheat and gluten free, high fibre

Kcals 270

Fat 13 g (2 g fat per 100 g)

Saturated fat 2 g

Sodium 210 mg

Fibre 5 g

Preparation time

25 minutes

Cooking time

about 40 minutes

Serves

4

NUTRITIONAL TIP

If you are on a dairy-free diet, stir in 300 ml (½ pint) extra stock instead of the milk. If eating wheat makes your symptoms worse, make sure you use wheat-free stock cubes or make your own stock with a chicken carcass.

carrot and chickpea soup

Quick and easy to make, this soup uses ingredients that you will probably already have in your storecupboard.

1 tablespoon sunflower oil

1 large onion, chopped

500 g (1 lb) carrots, diced

1 teaspoon ground cumin

1 teaspoon fennel seeds, roughly crushed

2 cm (¾ inch) root ginger, finely chopped

1 garlic clove, finely chopped

410 g (13¼ oz) can chickpeas, drained

1.2 litres (2 pints) gluten- and wheat-free vegetable stock

300 ml (½ pint) semi-skimmed milk

salt and pepper

GARNISH
40 g (1½ oz) flaked almonds

pinch of cumin powder

pinch of paprika

warm bread, to serve (optional)

1 Heat the oil in a medium-sized saucepan, add the onion and fry gently, stirring, for 5 minutes or until lightly browned. Mix in the carrots, ground spices, ginger and garlic and cook for 1 minute.

2 Mix in the chickpeas, stock and a little seasoning, bring to the boil, cover and simmer for 30 minutes or until the vegetables are tender.

3 Purée the soup in batches in a liquidizer or food processor until smooth then return to the pan and stir in the milk. Reheat gently.

4 Meanwhile, make the garnish. Heat the oil in a small frying pan, add the almonds, cumin and paprika and cook for 2–3 minutes until golden-brown. Ladle the soup into bowls and top with the almonds, cumin powder and paprika. Serve with warm bread, if liked.

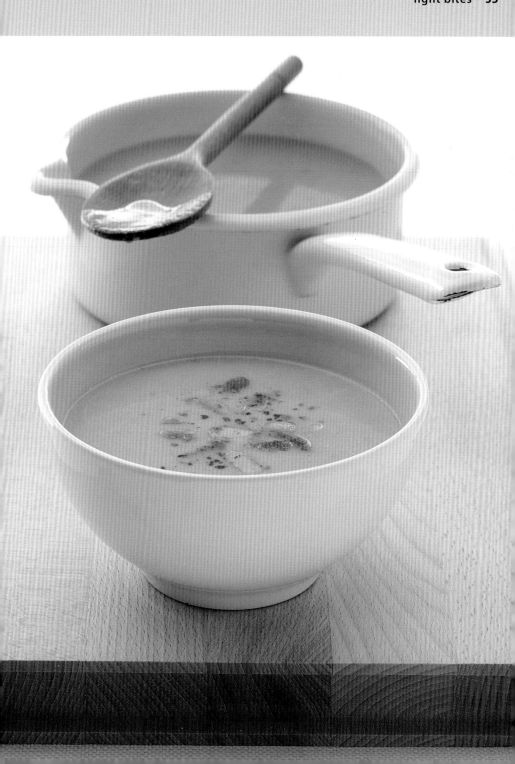

Nutrition

Wheat and gluten free, high fibre

Kcals 188

Fat 10 g

Saturated fat 4 g

Sodium 270 mg

Fibre 6 g

Preparation time

15 minutes

Cooking time

20 minutes

Serves

6

✚ **NUTRITIONAL TIP**

Peas are a good source of soluble fibre.

If you are serving this dish to vegetarians,

omit the bacon garnish.

green pea and coriander soup

Many people have a pack of frozen peas in the freezer, but how often do we use them for anything but a side dish? This quick and easy lunch is flavoured with coriander, but if you have some in the garden you might like to use mint instead.

1 tablespoon olive oil

1 onion, chopped

1 baking potato, about 200 g (7 oz), diced

1 litre (1¾ pints) gluten- and wheat-free vegetable stock

400 g (13 oz) frozen peas

about 25 g (1 oz) fresh coriander leaves

3 rashers of back bacon

6 tablespoons fromage frais

salt and pepper

1 Heat the oil in a heavy-based saucepan, add the onion and potato and fry gently, stirring, for 5 minutes or until softened but not browned.

2 Mix in the stock and a little seasoning. Bring to the boil, cover and simmer for 10 minutes. Add the peas and cook for 5 minutes until the vegetables are tender and the peas are still bright green.

3 Purée the soup in batches in a liquidizer or food processor until smooth, then return to the pan. Finely chop three-quarters of the coriander, stir into the soup and reheat.

4 Meanwhile, grill the bacon until crisp and then cut it into strips. Ladle the soup into bowls, add a spoonful of fromage frais to the top of each, lightly swirl into the soup and sprinkle with the bacon and remaining coriander leaves.

Nutrition
Gluten free, low fat
Kcals 39
Fat 1 g
Saturated fat 0 g
Sodium 465 mg
Fibre 2 g

Preparation time
10 minutes
Cooking time
9 minutes
Serves
4

NUTRITIONAL TIP
If you are not avoiding foods that contain wheat or gluten, you could use soy sauce instead of tamari sauce. If you are preparing this dish for vegetarians, check that the curry paste does not contain shrimp paste; also, omit the fish sauce and add a little lime juice instead.

oriental vegetable broth

There's no need to fry any of the vegetables first: simply add them to the flavoured stock and simmer for a few minutes. To make this more filling, you could add some finely diced cooked chicken breast or frozen prawns, which should be thawed first.

1 litre (1¾ pints) gluten-free vegetable stock

1–2 teaspoons red Thai curry paste (to taste)

1 tablespoon tamari sauce

2 teaspoons fish sauce (nam pla)

5 spring onions, thinly sliced

1 garlic clove, finely chopped

1 carrot, about 125 g (4 oz), thinly sliced

100 g (3½ oz) button mushrooms, thinly sliced

75 g (3 oz) broccoli, cut into tiny florets, stems sliced

50 g (2 oz) mangetout, sliced

small bunch of fresh coriander, torn into pieces

1 Put the stock, curry paste, tamari sauce and fish sauce into a saucepan. Add the white part of the spring onions, the garlic, sliced carrots and mushrooms and slowly bring to the boil. Reduce the heat and simmer for 5 minutes, stirring occasionally.

2 Add the broccoli and simmer for 2 minutes. Mix in the remaining green sliced spring onions, the mangetout and coriander leaves. Simmer for 2 minutes, then ladle the soup into bowls.

Nutrition

Low fat

Kcals 207

Fat 5 g

Saturated fat 1 g

Sodium 222 g

Fibre 3 g

Preparation time

10 minutes

Cooking time

10–12 minutes

Serves

4

NUTRITIONAL TIP

To increase the fibre levels in this dish, spread the wraps with hummus instead of the cheese or spoon the filling into warmed wholemeal pitta breads.

roasted vegetable wraps

Many people find raw peppers rather indigestible, but grilling and then skinning them solves the problem. Here the peppers are lightly flavoured with pesto, then wrapped with low-fat garlic and herb cheese and peppery rocket leaves for a tasty lunch.

1 red pepper, quartered, cored and deseeded

1 yellow or orange pepper, quartered, cored and deseeded

2 courgettes, about 300 g (10 oz) in total, sliced

4 teaspoons olive oil

1 teaspoon pesto

salt and pepper

4 large plain tortilla wraps

100 g (3½ oz) low-fat soft garlic and herb cheese

50 g (2 oz) rocket leaves

4 teaspoons balsamic vinegar

rocket salad, to garnish (optional)

1 Put the peppers on a foil-lined grill pan, skin side up, and arrange the courgettes around them in a single layer. Mix together the oil, pesto and a little seasoning and brush over the vegetables.

2 Cook under a preheated hot grill for 10–12 minutes, turning until the courgettes are lightly browned on both sides and the pepper skins are charred. Wrap the foil around the vegetables and set aside for 10 minutes.

3 Peel away and discard the softened skins from the peppers. Cut the pepper quarters and courgette slices into strips. Warm the wraps according to the directions on the packet, then spread the cheese in a strip down the centre of each wrap.

4 Top with the cooked vegetables, arrange the rocket leaves on the vegetables and drizzle with the vinegar. Roll up tightly, cut in half and serve immediately or wrap in clingfilm and eat later, with extra rocket salad, if liked.

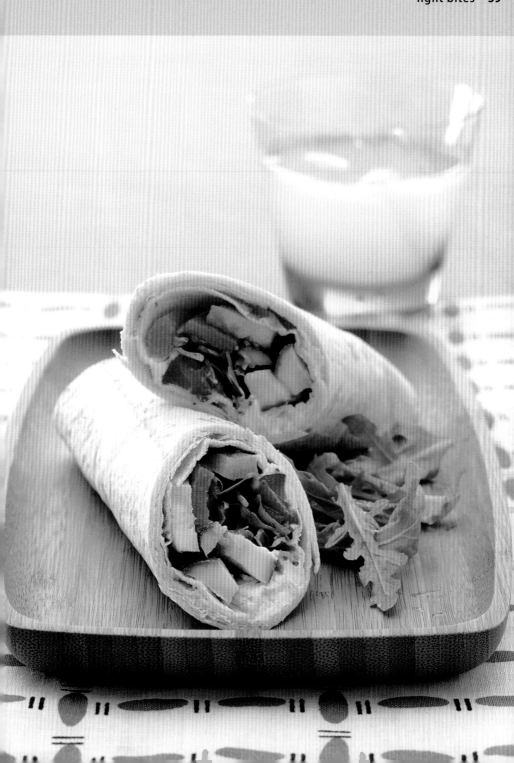

Nutrition
Wheat free, gluten free
Kcals 303
Fat 10 g
Saturated fat 3 g
Sodium 83 mg
Fibre 2 g

Preparation time
20 minutes
Cooking time
13–18 minutes
Serves
4

NUTRITIONAL TIP
Read the packet carefully when you are buying wasabi for the first time and make sure that it is gluten free. If you are on a low-fat diet, fromage frais is suitable because it has a very low fat content.

trout and new potato salad

Serve this salad while the potatoes and trout flakes are still warm; or, if you would rather make it in advance, leave the potatoes and trout to cool and toss with the dressing and salad leaves just before serving. Flaked smoked mackerel fillets would taste good in this salad but avoid those coated in peppercorns or the salad may be too fiery.

500 g (1 lb) baby new potatoes, scrubbed, larger ones halved

500 g (1 lb) trout fillets, rinsed and drained

150 g (5 oz) fromage frais

1–2 teaspoons gluten-free wasabi (Japanese horseradish), to taste

2 teaspoons set or clear honey

salt and pepper

100 g (3½ oz) salad leaves

1 Half-fill the base of a steamer with water and bring to the boil, add the potatoes to the water and put the fish fillets in a single layer in the steamer above. Cover and cook for 8 minutes until the fish is just cooked and flakes easily when pressed with a knife. Remove the top of the steamer, re-cover the potatoes, cook for 5–10 minutes more or until tender, then drain.

2 Transfer the fish to a plate or chopping board and break it into flakes, discarding the skin and any bones.

3 Mix the fromage frais with the wasabi, honey and a little seasoning in a salad bowl, add the warm potatoes and toss together. Add the fish flakes and salad leaves and toss together lightly. Serve immediately.

Nutrition

Dairy free, high fibre

Kcals 318

Fat 17 g

Saturated fat 2 g

Sodium 400 mg

Fibre 4 g

Preparation time

15 minutes

Cooking time

Serves

4

✚ **NUTRITIONAL TIP**

Couscous is made from Durum wheat, so, if you are avoiding wheat and foods that contain gluten, add cooked quinoa or millet grains instead.

couscous salad

Mix and match ingredients for this quick-to-put-together salad depending on what you have in the refrigerator. Canned or fresh salmon, diced cooked chicken, diced ham or crumbled feta could also be added instead of the tuna.

175 g (6 oz) couscous

450 ml (¾ pint) boiling water

200 g (7 oz) can tuna in spring water, drained

50 g (2 oz) sun-dried tomatoes, drained and thinly sliced

40 g (1½ oz) pitted black olives, roughly chopped

2 teaspoons capers, drained and roughly chopped (optional)

½ red onion, finely chopped

125 g (4 oz) cherry tomatoes, halved

50 g (2 oz) rocket or mixed salad leaves

DRESSING
3 tablespoons olive oil

juice of 1 lemon

small bunch of basil leaves, roughly torn

salt and pepper

1 Put the couscous in a bowl, pour over the boiling water and leave to soak for 5 minutes.

2 Flake the tuna into pieces and add them to the couscous with the sun-dried tomatoes, olives and capers (if used). Add the onion and cherry tomatoes and fork together.

3 Mix together the ingredients for the dressing, drizzle over the salad and lightly toss together. Sprinkle the salad leaves on top and serve.

Nutrition
Wheat, gluten and dairy free
Kcals 500
Fat 25 g
Saturated fat 4 g
Sodium 913 mg
Fibre 4 g

Preparation time
20 minutes
Cooking time
8–10 minutes
Serves
4

NUTRITIONAL TIP
Tamari sauce is the Japanese equivalent
of soy sauce and is wheat and gluten
free, but soy sauce can be used if you are
not avoiding wheat.

oriental salmon salad

Packed lunches needn't mean just sandwiches. This tasty rice salad can be made the
night before and taken to work in an insulated lunch box. Use a large can of salmon
instead of freshly grilled salmon if you prefer, and mangetout or sliced green beans
can be used instead of the sugar snap peas.

150 g (5 oz) long-grain rice

**4 salmon fillets, each about
125 g (4 oz)**

3 tablespoons tamari sauce

**100 g (3½ oz) sugar snap peas,
halved lengthways**

**1 large carrot, cut into
matchstick strips**

**4 spring onions, trimmed and
thinly sliced**

**100 g (3½ oz) bean sprouts,
rinsed and drained**

6 teaspoons sunflower oil

3 tablespoons sesame seeds

**2 teaspoons fish sauce
(nam pla) (optional)**

**2 teaspoons rice or white
wine vinegar**

**small bunch of fresh coriander
or basil, torn into pieces**

1 Half-fill a medium-sized saucepan with water and bring to
the boil. Add the rice to the water and simmer for 8 minutes.

2 Meanwhile, put the salmon on a foil-lined grill rack and
drizzle over 1 tablespoon of the tamari sauce. Cook under
a preheated grill for 8–10 minutes, turning once, until
browned and the fish flakes easily.

3 Add the sugar snap peas to the rice and cook for 1 minute.
Drain, rinse with cold water and drain again. Tip into a salad
bowl and mix in the carrot, spring onions and bean sprouts.

4 Heat 1 teaspoon oil in a nonstick frying pan, add the
sesame seeds and fry until just beginning to brown. Add
1 tablespoon of tamari sauce and quickly cover the pan so
that the seeds do not ping out. Take off the heat and leave
to stand for 1–2 minutes, then mix in the remaining tamari
sauce, oil, fish sauce (if used) and vinegar. Add the sesame
mixture to the salad and toss together. Take the skin off the
salmon and flake into pieces – discard any bones. Add to
the salad with the herb leaves and serve warm or cold.

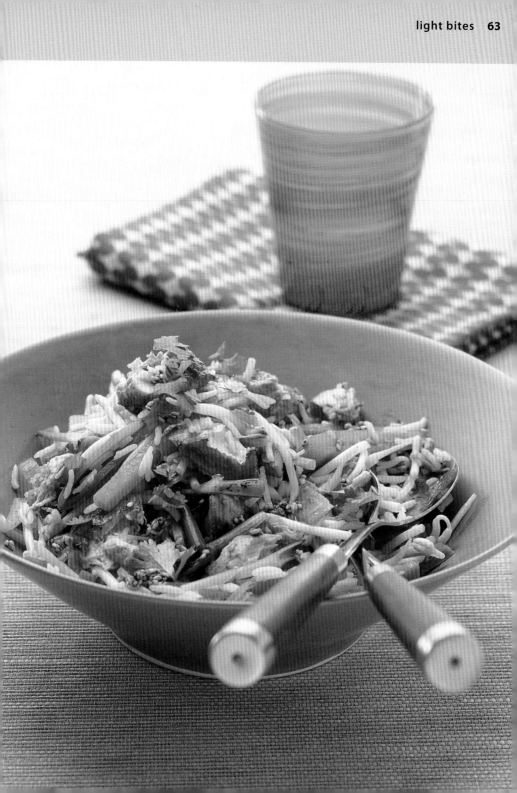

Nutrition

High fibre

Kcals 400

Fat 24 g

Saturated fat 7 g

Sodium 750 mg

Fibre 10 g

Preparation time

15 minutes

Cooking time

10–15 minutes

Serves

4

NUTRITIONAL TIP

Replace the feta cheese with tuna, salmon or chicken to make a dish suitable for a dairy-free diet.

white bean, feta and roasted pepper salad

This robust salad can be made in advance, so it's great for a healthy packed lunch. Take the salad leaves in a separate plastic bag to keep them crisp. The feta cheese could be omitted and a 185 g (6¼ oz) can of drained and flaked tuna in spring water included instead.

2 red peppers, halved, cored and deseeded

4 tablespoons olive oil

2 tablespoons balsamic or red wine vinegar

3 teaspoons sun-dried tomato paste

4 teaspoons capers, chopped if large

salt and pepper

2 x 410 g (13¼ oz) cans cannellini or haricot beans or chickpeas, drained

½ red onion, finely chopped

4 sticks celery, sliced

125 g (4 oz) feta cheese, drained

1 cos lettuce

1 Put the peppers, skin side up, on a foil-lined grill rack, brush with a little of the oil and cook under a preheated grill for 10–15 minutes until the peppers are softened and the skins charred. Wrap in foil and leave to cool.

2 Meanwhile, make the dressing by mixing the remaining oil with the vinegar, tomato paste, capers and seasoning.

3 Stir the drained beans or chickpeas, onion and celery into the dressing. Peel the skins off the peppers then cut the flesh into strips. Add to beans and gently toss together. Crumble the feta cheese over the top and serve the salad scooped over lettuce leaves.

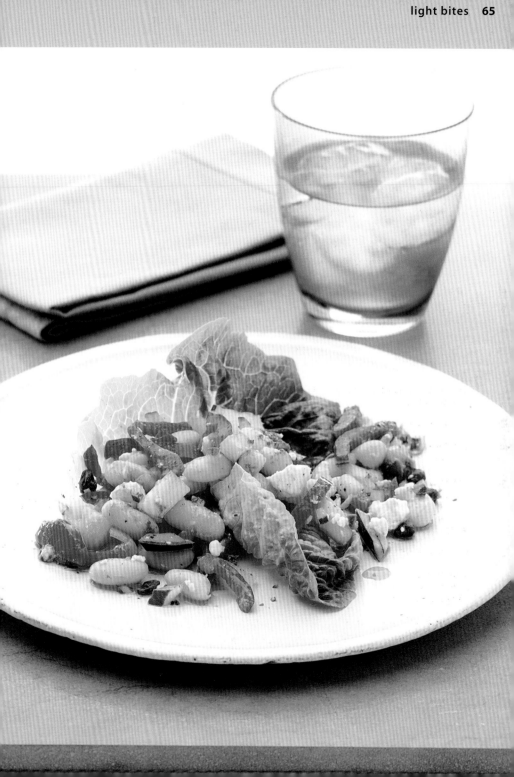

Nutrition
Gluten free, high fibre
Kcals 365
Fat 5 g (1 g fat per 100 g)
Saturated fat 3 g
Sodium 500 mg
Fibre 7 g

Preparation time
10 minutes
Cooking time
50–60 minutes
Serves
1

✚ **NUTRITIONAL TIP**
These fillings taste just as good served
with the traditional jacket potato. If
following a gluten-free diet, check that
the sweet chilli sauce and korma curry
paste are gluten free.

sweet potato with cottage cheese and chilli

We all love baked potatoes, but sweet potatoes make a lighter and more unusual
lunch choice and, for those avoiding wheat and gluten, a tasty and filling alternative
to sandwiches.

**1 sweet potato, about 300 g
(10 oz)**

100 g (3½ oz) cottage cheese

1 tablespoon sweet chilli sauce

few fresh coriander leaves

salt and pepper

1 Scrub and prick the sweet potato and cook it in a
preheated oven, 200°C (400°F), Gas Mark 6, for 50–60
minutes or until it is tender.

2 Cut the sweet potato in half then half again to make a
cross, fluff up the centre with a fork, then top with cottage
cheese, a little seasoning, a drizzle of chilli sauce and some
torn coriander leaves.

ALTERNATIVES
Curried ham Mix together 50 g (2 oz) low-fat natural yogurt
and 1 teaspoon korma curry paste in a small bowl. Stir in a
little red onion, finely chopped, and a 2 cm (¾ inch) thick
slice of cucumber, finely diced. Spoon over the top of
1 baked sweet potato (see above) and sprinkle with 1 large
slice of ham, roughly diced.

Avocado salsa Mix together in a bowl ½ ripe avocado,
stoned, peeled and diced, the juice of ½ lime, a little red
onion, finely chopped, ½ apple, cored and finely diced,
3 cherry tomatoes, quartered, and a few coriander leaves,
roughly chopped. Spoon the mixture over 1 baked sweet
potato (see above).

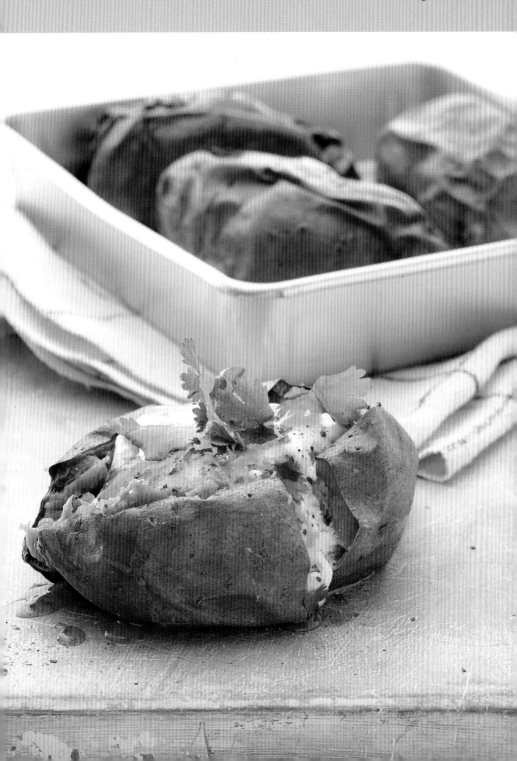

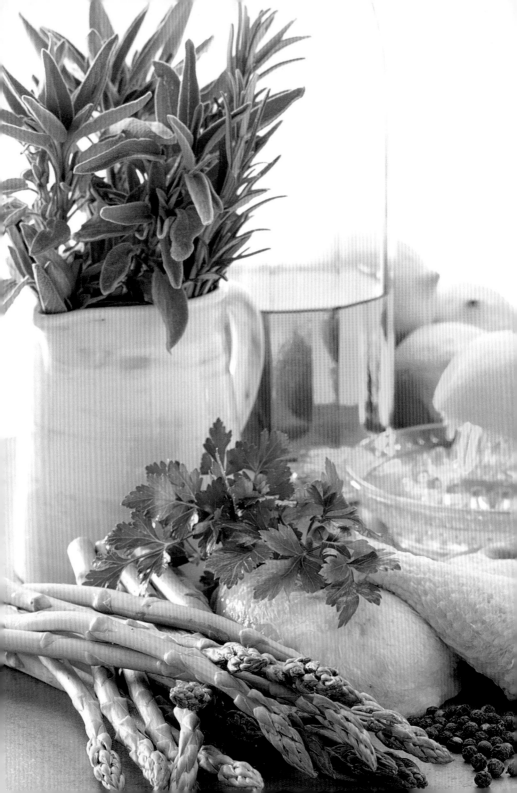

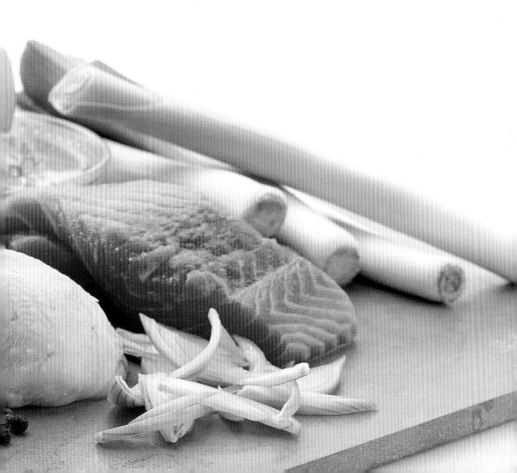

main
meals

Nutrition

Low fibre

Kcals 327

Fat 15 g

Saturated fat 4 g

Sodium 285 mg

Fibre 2 g

Preparation time

25 minutes

Cooking time

12–15 minutes

Serves

4

+ NUTRITIONAL TIP

The salsa can be used with other dishes if you are on a milk- or wheat-free diet.

sticky chicken with salsa

Refreshingly fruity, this dish makes a lovely summer supper. Cook the chicken under the grill or on the barbecue. The chicken can also be cut into cubes and threaded on to 8 skewers if you prefer. Use hot smoked Spanish pimento instead of paprika for a chilli-like oomph.

4 boneless, skinless chicken breasts, about 625 g (1¼ lb) in total

2 tablespoons tomato ketchup

1 tablespoon Worcestershire sauce

1 tablespoon sunflower oil

1 teaspoon Dijon mustard

1 teaspoon set or clear honey

½ teaspoon paprika

salt and pepper

green salad, to serve

new potatoes, to serve

SALSA
1 avocado, peeled and diced

1 small mango, peeled and diced

1 lime, grated rind and juice

2 tomatoes, skinned (if liked), deseeded and diced

½ small red onion, finely chopped

1 Rinse the chicken breasts with cold water, drain well, then put on a foil-lined grill rack.

2 Mix together the tomato ketchup, Worcestershire sauce, oil, mustard, honey, paprika and seasoning and brush over the chicken. Cook under a preheated grill for 12–15 minutes, turning several times, until the meat is browned and cooked through.

3 Meanwhile, make the salsa. Mix the diced avocado and mango with the lime rind and juice, then stir in the tomatoes and onion.

4 Slice the chicken into strips and transfer to plates. Serve with spoonfuls of salsa, with a green salad and some baby new potatoes.

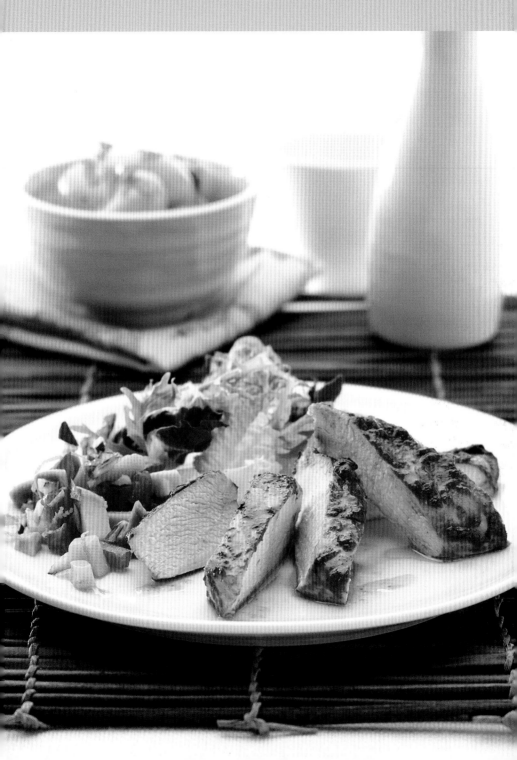

Nutrition

Dairy, wheat and gluten free

Kcals 372

Fat 13 g

Saturated fat 4 g

Sodium 636 mg

Fibre 9 g

Preparation time

20 minutes

Cooking time

about 2 hours

15 minutes

Serves

4

NUTRITIONAL TIP

Either pepperoni or chorizo can be used in this recipe, but read the labels carefully if you are avoiding wheat products to make sure that they are definitely wheat free because some makes contain wheat.

slow-cooked chicken

This all-in-one supper dish is ideal for weekends. You can prepare everything, then pop the casserole in the oven, leaving you free to garden or play with the children without fear of it spoiling.

1 tablespoon olive oil

8 chicken thighs, about 1 kg (2 lb) in total, skinned, boned and quartered

1 large onion, roughly chopped

1–2 garlic cloves, finely chopped

1 teaspoon hot smoked Spanish paprika (pimento)

400 g (13 oz) can chopped tomatoes

450 ml (¾ pint) wheat- and gluten-free chicken stock

410 g (13¼ oz) can borlotti beans, drained

salt and pepper

2–3 stems of rosemary

500 g (1 lb) baking potatoes, peeled and diced

2 carrots, about 250g (8 oz) in total, sliced

75 g (3 oz) pack sliced pepperoni

roughly chopped flat-leaf parsley, to garnish

1 Heat the oil in a large frying pan, add the chicken a few pieces at a time, until all the pieces have been added, then cook over a high heat for 5 minutes until lightly browned. Drain and transfer to a casserole dish.

2 Add the onion to the pan and cook, stirring, for 5 minutes or until pale golden. Add the garlic and paprika and cook, stirring, for 1 minute. Mix in the tomatoes, stock, beans, rosemary and seasoning and bring to the boil.

3 Add the potatoes, carrots and sliced pepperoni to the casserole dish, then pour over the hot tomato sauce. Cover and bake in a preheated oven, 180°C (350°F), Gas Mark 4, for 1½–2 hours until tender, adding a little extra stock if necessary. Spoon into bowls and serve sprinkled with parsley.

Nutritional value
Wheat free, gluten free
Kcals 560
Fat 24 g
Saturated fat 10 g
Sodium 235 mg
Fibre 4 g

Preparation time
20 minutes, plus
marinating
Cooking time
1 hour 40 minutes
Serves
4

NUTRITIONAL TIP
Cooking the potatoes in stock in a
separate dish rather than roasting them
around the meat makes a great low-fat
alternative to roast potatoes. You will also
need to strain any fat off the meat juices if
you serve these with the dish.

yogurt-marinated roast lamb

Inspired by East European cooking, this unusual way of roasting a leg of lamb keeps
it beautifully moist and full of flavour.

1.5–1.6 kg (3–3¼ lb) leg of lamb

2 garlic cloves, sliced

250 g (8 oz) low-fat natural yogurt

1 tablespoon olive oil

4 teaspoons chopped dill

1 teaspoon caraway seeds

1 teaspoon mild paprika

1 teaspoon black peppercorns, roughly crushed

salt

750 g (1½ lb) small baking potatoes, scrubbed

1 onion, sliced

1.8 litres (3 pints) hot wheat- and gluten-free lamb stock

15 g (½ oz) butter

1 Make slits at intervals over the lamb joint, cutting through
the fat into the meat, and insert a slice of garlic into each
slit. Transfer to a large non-metallic dish.

2 Mix together the yogurt, oil, dill, caraway, paprika,
peppercorns and salt and spread the mixture over the
lamb. Marinate for 3–4 hours in the refrigerator.

3 Put the lamb on a roasting rack in a roasting tin. Thinly
slice the potatoes and layer them in a shallow ovenproof
dish with the onion and a little extra seasoning. Pour in
600 ml (1 pint) hot stock. Dot the top with butter, cover
with foil and put on a high shelf in the oven.

4 Pour 600 ml (1 pint) hot stock into the roasting tin and
put the lamb under the potatoes in the oven. Roast in a
preheated oven, 190°C (375°F), Gas Mark 5, allowing
25 minutes per 500 g (1 lb) plus 25 minutes. Check on the
meat from time to time, and spoon stock over the lamb if it
looks dry or cover with foil if it is browning too quickly. Top
up the tin with extra stock as needed. Remove the foil from
the potatoes for the last 30 minutes of the cooking time.

5 Transfer the lamb to a warmed serving plate, then strain
the stock and meat juices from the tin into a jug. Serve with
the baked potatoes.

Nutrition
Wheat and gluten free, high fibre
Kcals 420
Fat 26 g
Saturated fat 7 g
Sodium 180 mg
Fibre 6 g

Preparation time
10 minutes
Cooking time
8–10 minutes
Serves
4

NUTRITIONAL TIP
Omit the lime juice and include soya yogurt instead of crème fraîche to make this dish suitable for a milk-free or an exclusion diet.

seared salmon with garden greens

The summery green vegetables in this dish require the same cooking time, but you could use broccoli, sugar snap peas, pak choi, spinach or any other vegetable you like. Make sure you put the vegetables that take the longest to cook in the steamer first.

4 salmon steaks, each about 150 g (5 oz), rinsed and dried

1 tablespoon olive oil

grated rind and juice of 1 lime

1 teaspoon set or clear honey

salt and pepper

250 g (8 oz) runner beans, stringed, cut into thin slices

250 g (8 oz) bunch of asparagus, trimmed, cut into 5 cm (2 inch) lengths

200 g (7 oz) frozen peas

6 tablespoons half-fat crème fraîche

4 teaspoons chopped mint

1 Put the salmon on a foil-lined grill rack. Mix together the oil, lime juice, honey and seasoning and spoon over both sides of the salmon. Grill the salmon under a preheated grill for 8–10 minutes, turning once, until it is browned on both sides and the fish flakes easily into even-coloured flakes when pressed with a knife.

2 Meanwhile, steam the runner beans, asparagus and frozen peas for 5 minutes. Mix the crème fraîche with the chopped mint, lime rind and a little seasoning.

3 Toss the just-cooked vegetables with the minted crème fraîche, spoon into the centre of 4 serving plates and arrange the salmon on top. Garnish with extra small mint leaves, if liked. Serve with new potatoes or rice.

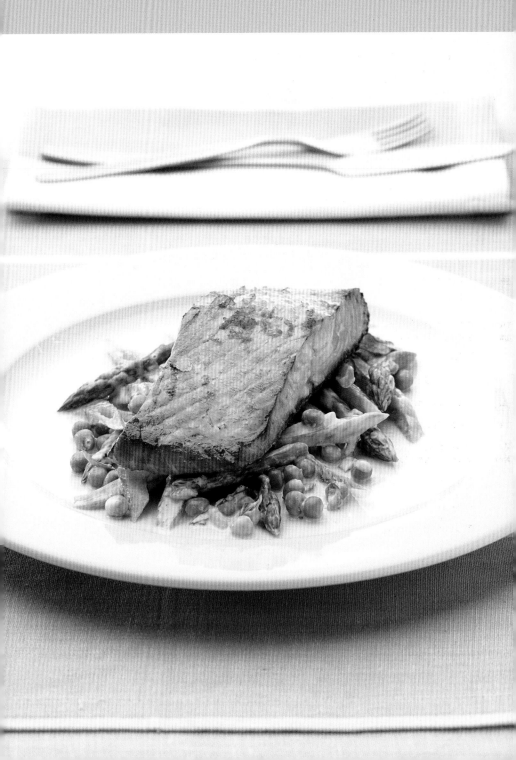

Nutrition
Wheat, gluten and dairy free
Kcals 593
Fat 31 g
Saturated fat 7 g
Sodium 1200 mg
Fibre 3 g

Preparation time
15 minutes
Cooking time
25–30 minutes
Serves
4

NUTRITIONAL TIP
Use white rice to make this dish suitable
for a low-fibre diet.

mixed fish kedgeree

If you have trouble persuading your family to adopt a healthier diet, this is a
good recipe to slip in. Because the brown rice is lightly spiced, they won't even
realize it is different.

1 onion, chopped

600 ml (1 pint) wheat- and
gluten-free fish or chicken
stock

200 g (7 oz) easy-cook
brown rice

½ teaspoon ground turmeric

5 cardamom pods, roughly
crushed

salt and pepper

300 g (10 oz) smoked haddock

300 g (10 oz) pack peppered or
plain smoked mackerel fillets

4 eggs, hard-boiled, shelled
and quartered

small bunch of fresh coriander

1 Put the onion, stock, rice, turmeric and cardamom pods
and the black seeds into a frying pan with a little seasoning.
Cut the haddock into 2 pieces and add them to pan. Bring
the stock to the boil, reduce the heat, cover and simmer for
10 minutes until the haddock is just cooked and flakes easily
into even-coloured flakes when pressed with a knife.

2 Lift the fish out of the pan, draining well, and transfer it to
a plate. Stir the rice then re-cover and simmer for 15–20
minutes until it is tender and most of the stock has been
absorbed by the rice. Stir several times towards the end of
cooking so that the rice does not stick to the pan.

3 Flake the smoked haddock into pieces, discarding the skin
and any bones. Do the same with the smoked mackerel. Stir
into the just-cooked rice, add the eggs and serve with torn
coriander leaves scattered over the top.

Nutrition
Wheat and gluten free, low fat
Kcals 357
Fat 16 g
Saturated fat 4 g
Sodium 278 mg
Fibre 2 g

Preparation time
15 minutes
Cooking time
30 minutes
Serves
4

NUTRITIONAL TIP
If you are avoiding dairy products, omit
the pesto and add some torn basil leaves
and a drizzle of olive oil to the chicken.

chicken en papillotte

Forget about lots of washing up, these tasty chicken parcels, flavoured with garlic,
pesto and sun-dried tomatoes, are baked in foil packets, which can be thrown
away after use.

**300 g (10 oz) baby new
potatoes, scrubbed and sliced**

150 g (5 oz) courgette, sliced

**100 g (3½ oz) mushrooms,
sliced**

**40 g (1½ oz) sun-dried
tomatoes in oil, drained and
sliced**

salt and pepper

**4 boneless, skinless chicken
breasts, each about 150 g (5 oz)**

4 teaspoons pesto

**2 small garlic cloves, finely
chopped (optional)**

½ small red onion, thinly sliced

**300 ml (½ pint) hot gluten- and
wheat-free chicken stock or red
or white wine**

**basil leaves, to garnish
(optional)**

1 Cook the potatoes in a small saucepan of boiling water for
5 minutes until just cooked. Drain.

2 Fold up the edges of 4 large pieces of foil to make
4 containers and put them in a large roasting tin. Spoon the
potatoes onto the foil and top with the courgette,
mushroom and tomato slices. Season lightly, then top each
with a chicken breast.

3 Add a teaspoon of pesto to the top of each chicken breast,
sprinkle with the garlic (if used) and red onion and pour the
stock around the chicken. Fold the foil over the top of the
chicken and twist the edges together to seal well.

4 Bake in a preheated oven, 220°C (425°F), Gas Mark 7, for
25 minutes or until the chicken is cooked through and the
juices run clear when pierced with a small knife. Transfer the
contents of the parcels to serving plates and serve garnished
with basil leaves, if liked.

Nutrition

Low fibre

Kcals 283

Fat 13 g

Saturated fat 3 g

Sodium 730 mg

Fibre 1 g

Preparation time

25 minutes

Cooking time

20–25 minutes

Serves

4

NUTRITIONAL TIP

Check the black olive pesto is milk free to enjoy this dish on a milk-free diet.

cod in Parma ham

This stylish-looking supper dish can be prepared in advance and kept in the refrigerator until you are ready to bake it.

2 cod loins, about 625 g (1¼ lb) in total, rinsed, drained and each halved crossways

juice of 1 lemon

salt and pepper

4 teaspoons black olive tapenade or black olive pesto

4 slices Parma ham, about 100 g (3½ oz) in total

1 tablespoon olive oil

1 small onion, finely chopped

1 garlic clove, finely chopped

500 g (1 lb) plum tomatoes, skinned, deseeded and diced or 400 g (13 oz) can chopped tomatoes

2 teaspoons sun-dried tomato paste

2 teaspoons balsamic vinegar (optional)

small bunch of basil

crusty bread, to serve

1 Drizzle the halved fish loins with lemon juice and season, then spread the top and sides with tapenade or pesto, avoiding the ends of the fish. Wrap the top and sides with ham, leaving the ends exposed.

2 Heat the oil in a saucepan, add the onion and garlic and fry for 5 minutes or until softened and lightly browned. Mix in the tomatoes, tomato paste, vinegar (if used) and seasoning. Tear the basil leaves into the sauce.

3 Spoon the sauce into a shallow, ovenproof dish and arrange the fish on top. Bake, uncovered, in a preheated oven, 190°C (375°F), Gas Mark 5, for 15 minutes until the ham has darkened slightly and the fish is pure white and flakes easily when pressed with a knife. Transfer to plates and serve with crusty bread and rice or new potatoes.

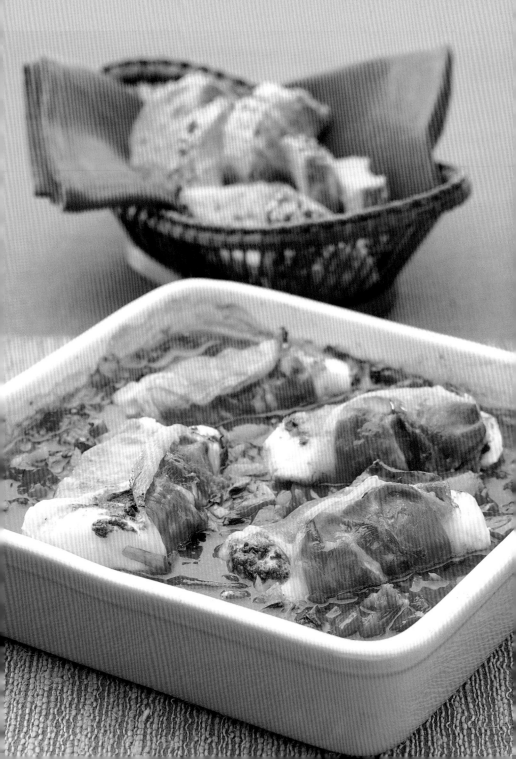

Nutrition
Wheat, gluten and dairy free
Kcals 315
Fat 10 g
Saturated fat 3 g
Sodium 114 mg
Fibre 4 g

Preparation time
15 minutes
Cooking time
2 hours
Serves
4

NUTRITIONAL TIP
Some people with IBS can find beef rather indigestible, but long, slow cooking seems to help. If you do have trouble with it, try not to eat red meat more than once a week and keep the portions small.

peppered beef

This hearty and warming supper can be put on to cook, leaving you free to do other things. If you get delayed the beef will still be fine after 2 hours.

1 tablespoon olive oil

625 g (1¼ lb) well-trimmed stewing beef, diced

1 onion, roughly chopped

1 garlic clove (optional)

2 tablespoons gluten- and wheat-free white bread flour

600 ml (1 pint) wheat- and gluten-free beef stock

1 tablespoon tomato purée

1 teaspoon juniper berries, roughly crushed

1 teaspoon peppercorns, roughly crushed

1 bay leaf

100 g (3½ oz) ready-to-eat prunes, pitted and halved

salt

1 Heat the oil in a large frying pan, add the beef, a few pieces at a time, until all the pieces have been added to the pan. Add the onion and fry, stirring, over a high heat until the meat is browned and the onion is just beginning to brown.

2 Stir in the garlic (if used) and the flour, then mix in the stock, tomato purée, juniper berries, peppercorns, bay leaf and prunes. Season with salt and bring to the boil, stirring.

3 Transfer the mixture to a casserole dish, cover and cook in a preheated oven, 160°C (325°F), Gas Mark 3, for 2 hours or until the beef is tender. Serve with sweet potato or celeriac mash and green beans.

Nutritional value
Gluten free, high fibre
Kcals 470
Fat 17 g
Saturated fat 7 g
Sodium 433 mg
Fibre 8 g

Preparation time
30 minutes
Cooking time
35 minutes
Serves
4

NUTRITIONAL TIP
If you prefer a thicker sauce, mix with a little water 1 tablespoon of cornflour or arrowroot and stir into the sauce at the end. If you are avoiding wheat and gluten, check the ingredients list on the mustard, stock cubes and cornflour before use.

hen house pie

Packed with moist pieces of chicken and lots of fresh vegetables, this pie is topped with cheesy leek and potato mash. It's a perfect supper to enjoy curled up in front of a film on television.

8 chicken thighs, about 1 kg (2 lb) in total

1 tablespoon olive oil

2 rashers of smoked back bacon, diced

2 leeks, about 200 g (7 oz) in total, thinly sliced

600 ml (1 pint) wheat- and gluten-free chicken stock

1 teaspoon Dijon mustard

2 tablespoons chopped sage

2 carrots, about 250 g (8 oz) in total, diced

salt and pepper

875 g (1¾ lb) potatoes, diced

200 g (7 oz) courgette, diced

100 g (3½ oz) frozen peas

4 tablespoons fromage frais

50 g (2 oz) mature Cheddar cheese, grated

1 Cut the skin away from the chicken thighs, cut the meat off the bones and cut it into chunks.

2 Heat the oil in a large frying pan, add the chicken a few pieces at a time until it has all been added, then add the bacon and white leek slices. Fry for 5 minutes, stirring until lightly browned. Add 450 ml (¾ pint) stock, the mustard, half the sage and the carrots. Season to taste, bring to the boil, cover and simmer for 25 minutes.

3 Meanwhile, cook the potatoes until tender, add the green leek slices and cook for 3 minutes more.

4 Add the courgettes, peas and remaining stock to the chicken mixture and simmer for 5 minutes. Transfer to a shallow, ovenproof dish.

5 Drain the potatoes and leeks and mash them with the fromage frais, remaining sage, half the cheese and seasoning. Spoon over the chicken mixture and sprinkle with the remaining cheese. Put under a preheated grill until the cheese is bubbling. Serve immediately.

Nutrition
High fibre, wheat free
Kcals 478
Fat 17 g
Saturated fat 6 g
Sodium 200 mg
Fibre 4 g

Preparation time
30 minutes
Cooking time
20 minutes
Serves
4

NUTRITIONAL TIP
Pork tenderloin is low in fat so is much
easier to digest than a more traditional
lamb or beef roast.

tamarind roasted pork

A stylish roast that is full of flavour. Tamarind has a distinctive, rather sour flavour, and
the paste is made from the dried pod of the tamarind tree, shaped into blocks. It is
used as a souring agent in many Southeast Asian dishes.

1 tablespoon olive oil

4 teaspoons tamarind paste

1 garlic clove, finely chopped

salt and pepper

4 pieces of pork tenderloin,
each 175 g (6 oz) and 10 cm
(4 inches) long

625 g (1¼ lb) sweet potato,
peeled, cut into chunks

2 tablespoons reduced-fat
crème fraîche

SALSA
1 dessert apple, cored, diced

½ red onion, finely chopped

½ teaspoon fennel seeds

2 tablespoons cider vinegar

1 teaspoon thick set or
clear honey

1 Put the oil, tamarind paste, garlic and seasoning in a plastic
bag, add the pieces of pork and toss together until the meat
is coated. Transfer to a roasting tin and cook in a preheated
oven, 190°C, 375°F, Gas Mark 5, for about 15 minutes until
browned and cook through.

2 Meanwhile, steam the sweet potato for 15–20 minutes or
until tender. Take the pork out of the oven, wrap it in foil and
leave to rest for 5 minutes.

3 Make the salsa. Place all the ingredients into a small
saucepan, cover and simmer for 3–4 minutes or until
warmed through.

4 Mash the sweet potato with the crème fraîche and a little
seasoning and spoon onto the centre of 4 serving plates.
Slice the pork thinly and arrange the slices on top of the
mash. Serve with green beans, a spoonful of the salsa with
the remainder in a small bowl and the meat juices from the
roasting tin drizzled around.

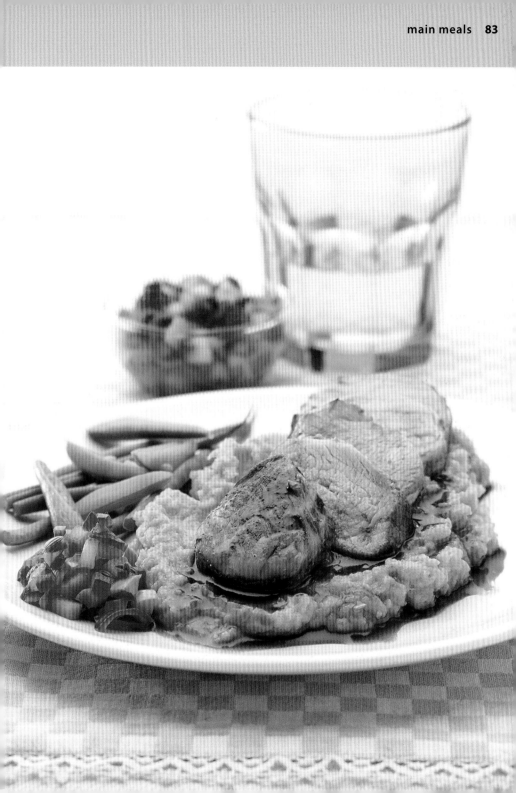

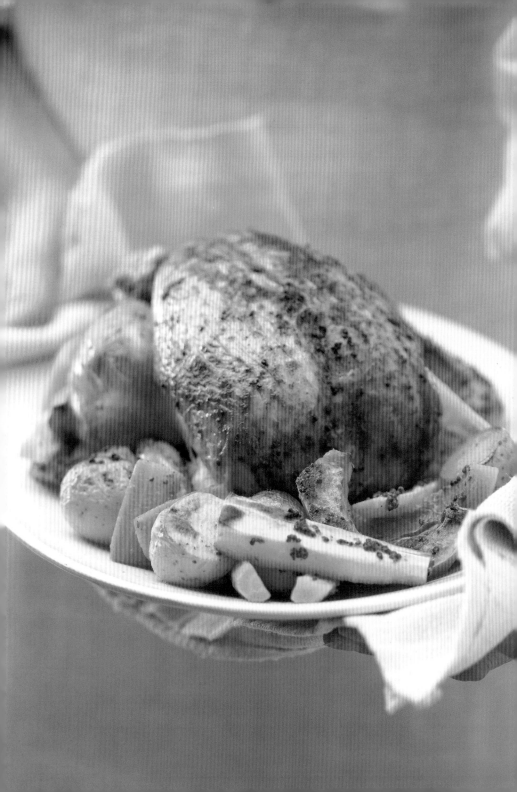

Nutrition
Wheat, gluten free and milk free
Kcals 610
Fat 34 g
Saturated fat 8 g
Sodium 270 mg
Fibre 6 g

Preparation time
25 minutes
Cooking time
1 hour 20 minutes
Serves
4

NUTRITIONAL TIP
Carefully read the label on the back of
the mustard and the stock cubes to
make sure that they really are gluten
free, because some brands may contain
wheat flour.

roasted mustard chicken

Glazing the chicken with a mix of honey, wholegrain mustard and spices means that
it cooks to a deep burnished gold. Serve the chicken on its own with the roasted
roots or accompany it with a steamed green vegetable.

1 chicken, about 1.5 kg (3 lb)

3 tablespoons sunflower oil

2 teaspoons wholegrain mustard

2 teaspoons clear honey

½ teaspoon turmeric

½ teaspoon paprika

salt and pepper

½ butternut squash, about 300 g (10 oz), peeled and deseeded

3 carrots, about 300 g (10 oz) in total

2 parsnips, about 250 g (8 oz) in total

300 g (10 oz) baby new potatoes, scrubbed

300 ml (½ pint) chicken or vegetable stock

1 Rinse the chicken inside and out with cold water, drain
well and transfer to a large roasting tin.

2 Mix the oil, mustard, honey, spices and seasoning together
in a large mixing bowl, then brush a little over the chicken.
Loosely cover with oiled foil and roast in a preheated oven,
190°C, 375°F, Gas Mark 5, for 30 minutes.

3 Meanwhile, cut the flesh of the butternut squash into thick
slices. Cut the carrots and parsnips into chunky sticks. Halve
any large potatoes.

4 Remove the foil from the chicken and brush with some
more mustard mixture. Add the vegetables to the remaining
mustard mix and toss together in the bowl. Spoon around
the chicken and roast for 50 minutes, turning once or twice
and re-covering the chicken after 20–30 minutes or when
the skin is deep brown.

5 Insert a skewer through the thickest part of the chicken leg
into the breast. If the juices run clear, transfer the chicken and
vegetables to a serving plate. If not, return to the oven and
retest after 15 minutes. Pour off half the fat from the roasting
tin, add the stock to the remaining juices, bring to the boil,
and strain into a jug before serving.

Nutrition	Preparation time	NUTRITIONAL TIP
Wheat free, gluten free	15 minutes	If you are on a dairy-free diet, omit the
Kcals 319	**Cooking time**	Greek yogurt altogether or use soya
Fat 18 g	about 1 hour	yogurt instead.
Saturated fat 8 g	10 minutes	
Sodium 185 mg	**Serves**	
Fibre 3 g	4	

spicy lamb with aubergine

This dish has all the flavour of a Greek moussaka but none of the fiddle. If you prefer not to serve it with rice, it would taste delicious topped with mashed potato mixed with fromage frais rather than butter and milk and browned in the oven.

1 tablespoon olive oil

1 onion, chopped

500 g (1 lb) lean lamb, minced

1 aubergine, about 250 g (8 oz), halved lengthways and thinly sliced

1–2 garlic cloves, finely chopped

400 g (13 oz) can chopped tomatoes

1 teaspoon ground cinnamon

¼ teaspoon grated nutmeg

300 ml (½ pint) wheat- and gluten-free lamb or chicken stock

salt and pepper

4 tablespoons Greek yogurt, to serve

roughly chopped mint or flat-leaf parsley, to serve

paprika (optional)

1 Heat the oil in a flameproof casserole, add the onion and lamb and fry for 2 minutes. Add the aubergine and fry for 5 minutes or until the lamb is evenly browned and the onion and aubergine are softened.

2 Stir in the garlic, tomatoes, spices, stock and a little seasoning. Bring to the boil, stirring, and cover.

3 Cook the lamb mixture in a preheated oven, 180°C (350°F), Gas Mark 4, for 1 hour or until tender. Serve with rice and topped with a spoonful of Greek yogurt and a sprinkling of mint, parsley and paprika, if liked.

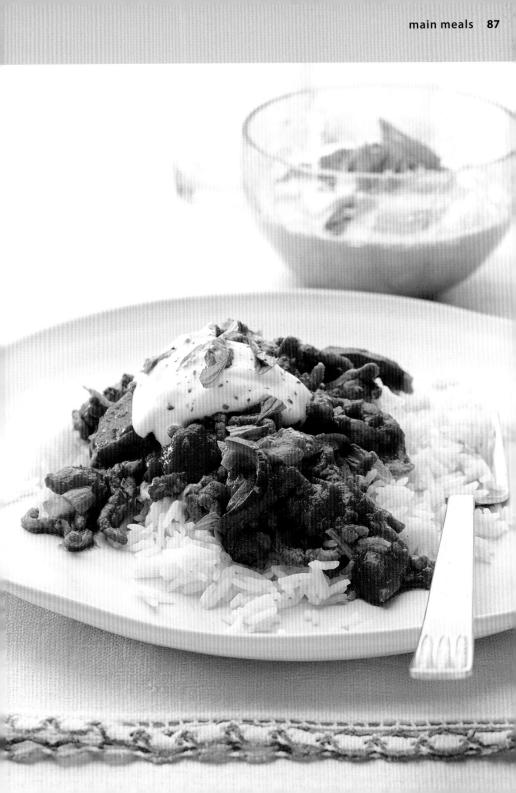

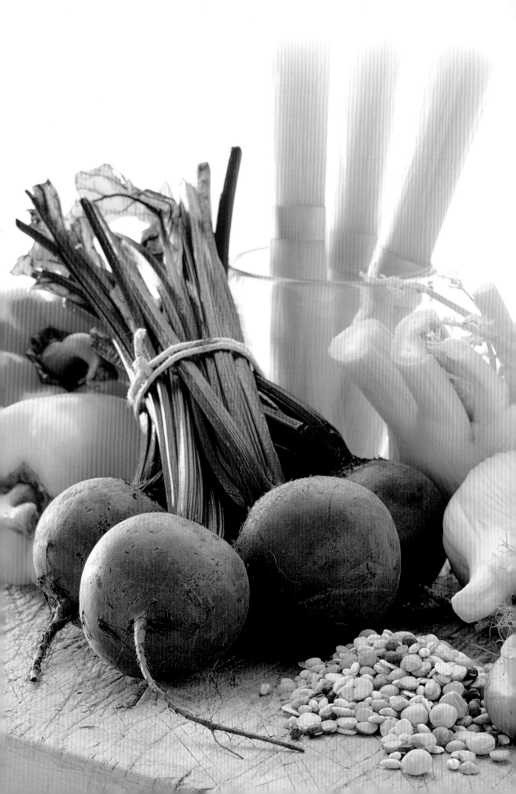

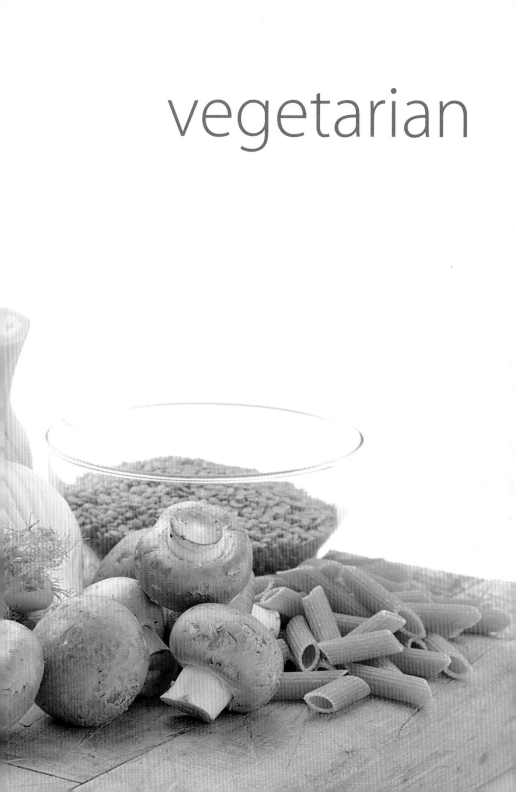

vegetarian

Nutrition
Wheat and gluten free, high fibre
Kcals 380
Fat 15 g
Saturated fat 7 g
Sodium 357 mg
Fibre 4 g

Preparation time
15 minutes
Cooking time
about 30 minutes
Serves
4

NUTRITIONAL TIP
If you cannot tolerate dairy products, omit
the cheese. Check that the cheese you are
using is suitable for vegetarians and is not
made with rennet.

beetroot and blue cheese risotto

A vibrant red, soft and creamy risotto is speckled with just-melting blue cheese.
Serve as soon as the rice is cooked or the liquid will quickly be absorbed because the
rice swells on standing. If you're not a fan of blue cheese, add a little freshly grated
Parmesan instead.

1 tablespoon olive oil

1 onion, finely chopped

3 small uncooked beetroot,
trimmed weight about 375 g
(12 oz), peeled and diced

200 g (7 oz) arborio rice

salt and pepper

few sage leaves, plus extra
to garnish

1.2 litres (2 pints) hot wheat-
and gluten-free vegetable
stock

125 g (4 oz) St Agur, Stilton
or other blue cheese, rind
removed, and diced

1 Heat the oil in a nonstick frying pan, add the onion and fry
gently, stirring occasionally, for 5 minutes or until softened.
Stir in the beetroot and cook for 2 minutes.

2 Stir in the rice, then add the sage, a little seasoning and
about one-third of the hot stock. Simmer, uncovered, for
15–20 minutes until the rice is soft and creamy and the
beetroot is tender, topping up with the remaining stock and
stirring more frequently towards the end of cooking.

3 Stir in the cheese and sprinkle with extra sage leaves,
if liked. Spoon into bowls and serve immediately.

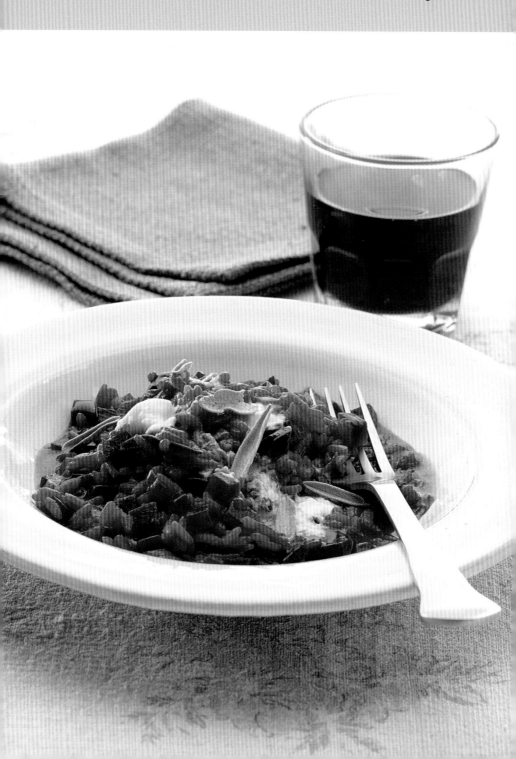

Nutrition
Wheat, gluten and dairy free
Kcals 340
Fat 13 g
Saturated fat 3 g
Sodium 513 mg
Fibre 4 g

Preparation time
20 minutes
Cooking time
about 30 minutes
Serves
4

NUTRITIONAL TIP
The fibre content of the dish will vary depending on the vegetable you choose and the type of rice. To reduce the fibre level, use white rice.

special fried rice

Popular with all ages, this tasty supper can be made with whatever vegetables you have in the refrigerator. Just take care that you cut them into small pieces so that they cook quickly.

200 g (7 oz) easy-cook brown rice

3 eggs

1 tablespoon water

salt and pepper

6 teaspoons sunflower oil

4 spring onions, sliced

125 g (4 oz) courgette, diced

½ red pepper, cored, deseeded and diced

50 g (2 oz) mangetout, sliced

75 g (3 oz) frozen peas

2.5 cm (1 inch) root ginger, peeled and grated

2 tablespoons sesame seeds

2 tablespoons tamari sauce

1 Cook the rice in boiling water for about 25 minutes or according to the instructions on the packet until just tender.

2 Meanwhile, beat together the eggs, water and a little seasoning in a bowl. Heat 2 teaspoons oil in a large frying pan, add the eggs and make a thin omelette. When the underside is golden, turn it over and cook the other side for a minute more. Slide it out of pan on to a plate and set aside.

3 Heat 3 teaspoons oil in the frying pan, add the spring onions, courgette, red pepper, mangetout, peas and ginger. Stir fry for 3–4 minutes or until tender. Drain the rice, tip it back into the dried pan and stir in the stir-fried vegetables.

4 Heat the remaining oil in a frying pan, add the sesame seeds and fry for 2–3 minutes, stirring until just beginning to brown. Turn off the heat, add the tamari sauce and quickly cover the pan so that the seeds do not ping out.

5 Roll up the omelette, cut it into thin slices and add to the rice with the sesame seeds. Spoon into bowls and serve.

Nutrition
Wheat and gluten free, high fibre
Kcals 533
Fat 16 g
Saturated fat 2 g
Sodium 860 mg
Fibre 4 g

Preparation time
15 minutes
Cooking time
8–10 minutes
Serves
4

NUTRITIONAL TIP
Use soya yogurt in the tzatziki to make
this dish suitable for a dairy-free diet.

falafel

These chickpea patties are traditionally deep-fried, but this shallow-fried version
is healthier. Made in minutes using a can of chickpeas, falafel are packed with
protein and fibre.

1 onion, quartered

small bunch of parsley or chives

2 garlic cloves, sliced

2 x 410 g (13¼ oz) cans
chickpeas, drained

2 teaspoons cumin seeds,
finely crushed

2 teaspoons coriander seeds,
finely crushed

1 teaspoon wheat- and gluten-
free baking powder

3 tablespoons olive oil

salt and pepper

TZATZIKI
100 g (3½ oz) cucumber,
finely diced

150 g (5 oz) low-fat natural
yogurt

few fresh mint leaves

4 pitta breads, to serve

2 Little Gem lettuce leaves,
to serve

1 Put all the ingredients for the falafel into a food processor
and blend to make a coarse, thick purée. Alternatively,
liquidize in batches or finely chop the onion, herbs, garlic
and chickpeas and mix them with the remaining
ingredients.

2 Use 2 dessertspoons to shape the mixture into 16 oval
patties. Heat 1 tablespoon oil in a large, nonstick frying pan,
add half the falafel and fry for 4–5 minutes, turning until
golden and crisp on the outside and piping hot. Add extra
oil if needed. Repeat with the remaining falafel.

3 Meanwhile, make the tzatziki by mixing together the
ingredients in a bowl. Warm the pitta breads under the grill
and shred the lettuce if liked. Arrange on serving plates
with the hot falafel.

Nutrition
Wheat and gluten free, high fibre
Kcals 285
Fat 10 g
Saturated fat 4 g
Sodium 413 mg
Fibre 5 g

Preparation time
25 minutes
Cooking time
about 1 hour
10 minutes
Serves
4

✚ **NUTRITIONAL TIP**
If you are avoiding wheat and gluten and
are not on a dairy-free diet, omit the toast
and add some sliced cheese once the
ratatouille has been served. You could also
serve this with baked potato, rice or pasta.

oven-baked ratatouille

Florence fennel adds a delicate aniseed flavour to this rich ratatouille, which is
speckled with peppers and courgettes and topped with toasted baguette slices
and creamy, just-melting goats' cheese with chives.

1 tablespoon olive oil

1 onion, chopped

2 garlic cloves, finely chopped

1 fennel bulb, about 250 g
(8 oz), diced

3 coloured peppers, cored,
deseeded and diced

2 courgettes, about 300 g
(10 oz) in total, diced

400 g (13 oz) can chopped
tomatoes

150 ml (¼ pint) wheat- and
gluten-free vegetable stock

1 teaspoon caster sugar

salt and pepper

rocket salad, to serve

TOPPING
1 baguette, about 150 g (5 oz)
in total, thinly sliced

125 g (4 oz) goats' cheese
with chives

1 Heat the oil in a large, nonstick frying pan. Add the onion
and fry, stirring, for 5 minutes or until lightly browned. Add
the garlic and remaining fresh vegetables and fry for a further
2 minutes.

2 Stir in the canned tomatoes, stock, sugar and a little
seasoning. Bring to the boil, stirring, then transfer to a deep
ovenproof dish. Cover the top of the dish with foil and bake
in a preheated oven, 190°C (375°F), Gas Mark 5, for 45–60
minutes until the vegetables are tender.

3 When the vegetables are almost ready, grill one side of
the bread slices. Slice the cheese and add one slice to each
untoasted side of bread. Remove the foil from the ratatouille,
stir the vegetables and top with the toasts, cheese side up.

4 Put the ratatouille under a preheated grill for 4–5 minutes
until the cheese is just beginning to melt. Spoon into shallow
bowls and serve with a rocket salad.

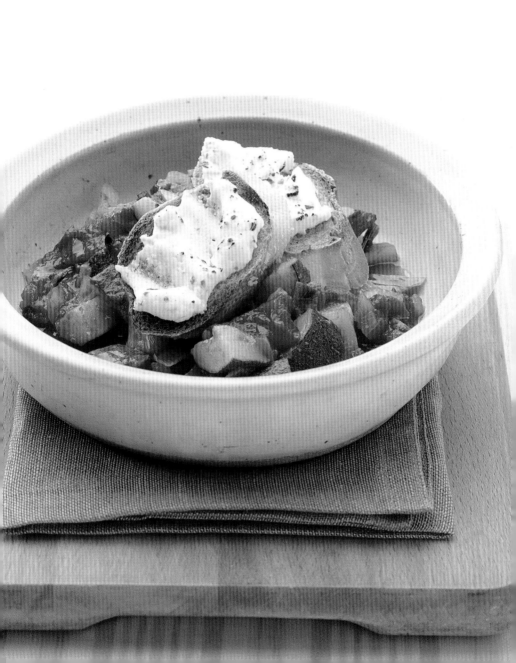

Nutrition
Dairy free, high fibre
Kcals 305
Fat 5 g
Saturated fat 1 g
Sodium 47 mg
Fibre 5 g

Preparation time
15 minutes
Cooking time
30 minutes
Serves
4

NUTRITIONAL TIP
Spicy foods can upset IBS. Choosing milder spices or cutting the amount used may help.

bulgar pilaf with mixed roots

An easy store cupboard supper, this can be served as it is or topped with spoonfuls of yogurt, toasted nuts or torn mint or parsley leaves. Cut the vegetables into small dice so that they cook quickly.

1 tablespoon olive oil

1 red onion, sliced

150 g (5 oz) parsnip, diced

200 g (7 oz) carrot, diced

250 g (8 oz) swede, diced

4 cloves

1 teaspoon ground cinnamon

1 teaspoon mild paprika

½ teaspoon ground cumin

410 g (13¼ oz) can green lentils, drained

125 g (4 oz) bulgar wheat

1 tablespoon tomato purée

salt and pepper

900 ml (1½ pint) vegetable stock

1 Heat the oil in a large, nonstick frying pan, add the onion and fry, stirring, for 5 minutes or until softened. Stir in the root vegetables and fry for 2 minutes.

2 Mix in the spices, cook for a further minute, then add the lentils, bulgar wheat, tomato purée and a little seasoning. Pour in 600 ml (1 pint) stock and bring to the boil.

3 Reduce the heat, cover and simmer for 20 minutes, stirring and topping up with extra stock as needed, until the vegetables are tender. Spoon into bowls to serve.

Nutrition

Wheat, gluten and dairy free

Kcals 389

Fat 20 g

Saturated fat 8 g

Sodium 614 g

Fibre 2 g

Preparation time

10 minutes

Cooking time

10 minutes

Serves

4

NUTRITIONAL TIP

The fibre content of this dish will depend on the vegetables you use, so you can adjust the recipe for either a high- or a low-fibre diet.

mixed vegetable and cashew laska

This light, refreshing and colourful curry can be cooked in under 10 minutes. Vary the vegetables depending on what you have in the refrigerator.

125 g (4 oz) medium rice noodles

2 teaspoons sunflower oil

1 onion, finely chopped

75 g (3 oz) cashew nuts

2 teaspoons wheat- and gluten-free red Thai curry paste

1 garlic clove, finely chopped

400 ml (14 fl oz) can reduced-fat coconut milk

300 ml (½ pint) wheat- and gluten-free vegetable stock

100 g (3½ oz) carrot, cut into matchstick strips

1 red pepper, cored, deseeded and diced

50 g (2 oz) mangetout, sliced

100 g (3½ oz) pak choi, sliced

2 tablespoons tamari sauce

small bunch of basil or fresh coriander

1 Cook the noodles in boiling water according to the instructions on the packet.

2 Meanwhile, heat the oil in a wok or second saucepan, add the onion and cashew nuts and fry for 3–4 minutes until just beginning to brown. Stir in the curry paste and garlic, then mix in the coconut milk and stock.

3 Bring the coconut broth to the boil, add the carrot and red pepper and simmer for 3 minutes. Mix in the mangetout and pak choi and cook for a further 2 minutes until the leaves have just wilted. Stir in the tamari sauce and half the basil or coriander, torn into pieces.

4 Drain the noodles and stir them into the coconut broth. Spoon into bowls and top with the remaining basil or coriander leaves.

Nutrition
High fibre
Kcals 404
Fat 11 g
Saturated fat 3 g
Sodium 33 mg
Fibre 11 g

Preparation time
15 minutes
Cooking time
15 minutes
Serves
4

NUTRITIONAL TIP
Reduce the fat content even more by using low-fat ricotta or quark cheese instead of the crème fraîche. If you are avoiding dairy products, omit the crème fraîche altogether.

penne with roasted tomatoes

Wholewheat pasta has been used here, but plain pasta or corn pasta can be used instead. Alternatively, spoon the tomato sauce over the top of a baked potato.

500 g (1 lb) cherry tomatoes, halved

2 tablespoons olive oil

2 garlic cloves, finely chopped

4–5 stems rosemary

large pinch of smoked paprika or chilli powder

salt and pepper

375 g (12 oz) dried wholewheat pasta twists or tubes

2 tablespoons balsamic vinegar

4 tablespoons reduced-fat crème fraîche

Parmesan shavings, to serve

1 Put the tomatoes in a roasting tin, drizzle with the oil and sprinkle with the garlic, torn leaves from 3 rosemary stems, the paprika or chilli powder and a little seasoning. Roast in a preheated oven, 200°C (400°F), Gas Mark 6, for 15 minutes until just softened.

2 Meanwhile, cook the pasta in a large saucepan of boiling water for 10–12 minutes or until just tender, then drain.

3 Spoon the balsamic vinegar into the tomatoes, add the drained pasta and crème fraîche and lightly toss together. Spoon into bowls and top with Parmesan shavings.

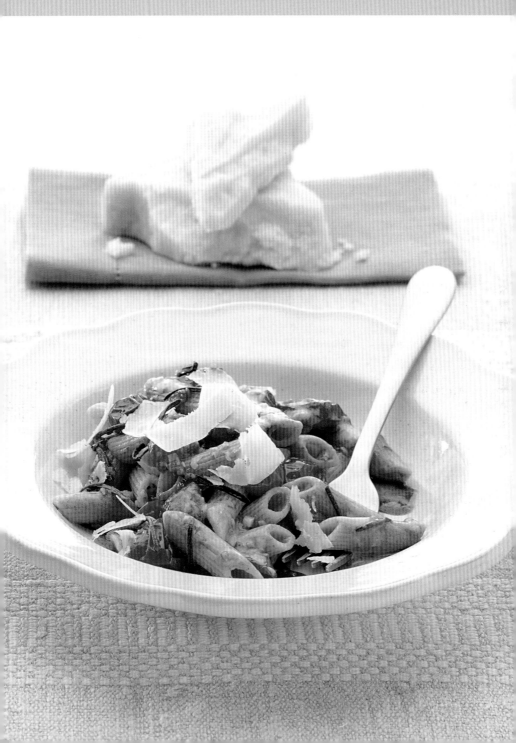

Nutrition

Wheat, gluten and dairy free

Kcals 186

Fat 12 g

Saturated fat 3 g

Sodium 118 mg

Fibre 1 g

Preparation time

10 minutes

Cooking time

12–14 minutes

Serves

4

NUTRITIONAL TIP

Increase the fibre levels by adding frozen peas or frozen broad beans together with the diced courgette.

minted courgette frittata

A quick and easy storecupboard summer supper, this is even easier if you have fresh mint growing in your garden. If you don't have any fresh herbs use a little chopped watercress or rocket leaves or some frozen parsley. If you like, add some diced chorizo, bacon, salami or ham or extra vegetables when you fry the courgettes.

4 teaspoons olive oil

1 red onion, thinly sliced

375 g (12 oz) courgette, diced

6 eggs

2 tablespoons water

2 tablespoons chopped mint

salt and pepper

mixed salad, to serve

1 Heat 3 teaspoons oil in a large, nonstick frying pan, add the onion and courgettes and fry over a gentle heat for 5 minutes or until lightly browned and just cooked.

2 Beat the eggs, water, chopped mint and a little seasoning together. Heat the remaining oil in the frying pan and pour in the egg mixture. Cook, without stirring, for 4–5 minutes or until the frittata is almost set and the underside is golden-brown.

3 Transfer the pan to a hot grill (making sure that the handle is away from the heat) and cook for 3–4 minutes until the top is golden and the frittata is cooked through. Cut into wedges or squares and serve with a mixed salad.

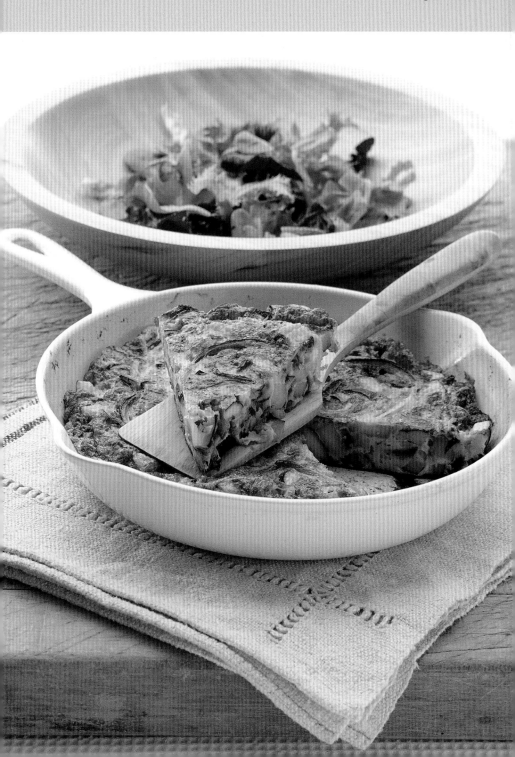

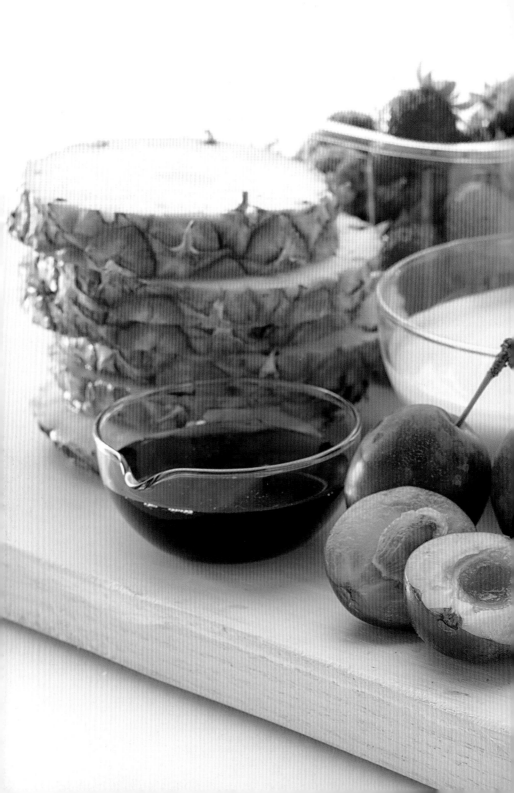

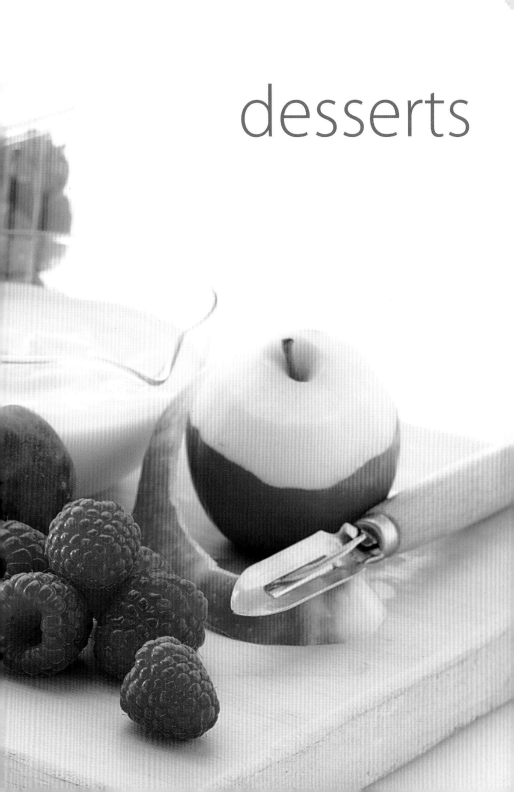

desserts

Nutrition
Wheat and gluten free, low fibre
Kcals 125
Fat 2 g (1 g fat per 100 g)
Saturated fat 1 g
Sodium 33 mg
Fibre 2 g

Preparation time
15 minutes
Cooking time
15 minutes
Serves
4

NUTRITIONAL TIP
If you are not on a dairy-free diet, serve the peaches with scoops of vanilla ice cream. Make sure you use chocolate with 70 per cent cocoa solids if you are avoiding milk and check the ingredients list to make sure it is dairy free.

peach melba meringues

When you're short of time but really want to make a pudding to impress your friends, this is the answer. Halved and baked peaches are topped with a square of melting chocolate and a soft-centred marshmallow meringue topping before being drizzled with a ruby-red fresh raspberry sauce.

2 large peaches, halved and pitted

4 squares of dark chocolate, about 25 g (1 oz)

2 egg whites

50 g (2 oz) caster sugar

200 g (7 oz) raspberries (just thawed if frozen)

a little sifted icing sugar, to decorate (optional)

1 Put the peaches, cut side up, in a shallow ovenproof dish, add 2 tablespoons water to the base of the dish and cover the peaches loosely with foil. Bake in a preheated oven, 180°C (350°F), Gas Mark 4, for 10 minutes.

2 Add a square of chocolate to the centre of each peach half, re-cover and return to the oven.

3 Meanwhile, make the meringue. Whisk the egg whites until they form stiff but moist-looking peaks. Gradually whisk in the sugar, a teaspoonful at a time, until the mixture is thick and glossy.

4 Spoon the meringue over the peaches and swirl into peaks with the back of the spoon. Return the peaches to the oven for 5–7 minutes until the meringue is cooked through and the swirls are tinged with brown.

5 Meanwhile, purée 125 g (4 oz) of the raspberries and sieve to remove the seeds. Transfer the peaches to serving plates, decorate with the remaining whole raspberries, drizzle the sauce around and dust with sifted icing sugar, if liked. Serve immediately.

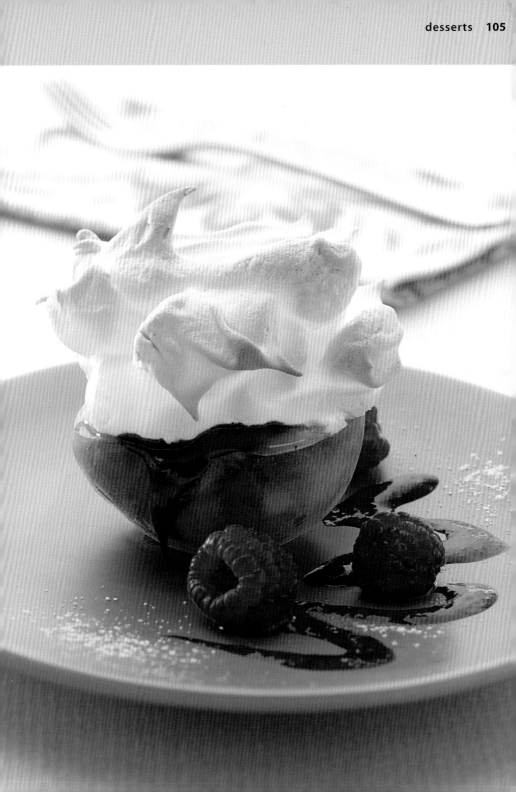

Nutrition
Wheat, gluten and dairy free
Kcals 249
Fat 9 g
Saturated fat 6 g
Sodium 120 mg
Fibre 3 g

Preparation time
20–30 minutes, plus
freezing
Cooking time
none
Serves
4

NUTRITIONAL TIP
This is much lower in sugar and fat than
a more conventional dairy ice cream.

lychee and coconut ice

This dairy-free ice cream tastes delicious when it is used to sandwich tiny pairs of spooned or piped meringues. If you make the ice cream in advance, leave it at room temperature for about 15 minutes to soften slightly before scooping.

425 g (14 oz) can lychees in natural syrup

50 g (2 oz) icing sugar

grated rind of 2 limes

400 ml (14 fl oz) can reduced-fat coconut milk

500 g (1 lb) strawberries

1 Put the lychees and the juice into a liquidizer or food processor, reserving 2 for decoration later. Add the icing sugar and purée until smooth.

2 Stir in the lime rind and coconut milk, then pour into a chilled ice-cream maker and churn until thick enough to scoop, which should take about 30 minutes. Alternatively, pour the mixture into a shallow stainless-steel roasting tin and freeze for 4–6 hours, beating 2–3 times with a fork or blitzing in a food processor to break down the ice crystals and returning to the freezer until it is firm enough to scoop.

3 Meanwhile, hull and purée half the strawberries. Sieve to remove the seeds. Slice or quarter the remaining fruits, depending on their size.

4 To serve, scoop the coconut ice into glasses, drizzle with the puréed sauce and top with the remaining berries and reserved lychees, cut into slices.

Nutrition

Wheat and gluten free, low fat

Kcals 197

Fat 5 g

Saturated fat 3 g

Sodium 68 mg

Fibre 3 g

Preparation time

30 minutes

Cooking time

45 minutes

Serves

4

NUTRITIONAL TIP

Some brands of cornflour contain wheat flour, so read the ingredients list carefully if you are avoiding gluten. To make this suitable for a milk-free diet, use soya cream or yogurt.

brown sugar pavlovas with berries

Don't wait for a special occasion to make this dish. Serve four now and leave the plain pavlovas in an airtight tin for up to three days, then just top them with fresh, frozen or canned fruit as and when you need them.

3 egg whites

100 g (3½ oz) soft light muscovado sugar

75 g (3 oz) caster sugar

1 teaspoon gluten-free cornflour

1 teaspoon white wine vinegar

TO DECORATE
200 ml (7 fl oz) reduced-fat crème fraîche

150 g (5 oz) raspberries (just thawed if frozen)

250 g (8 oz) strawberries, sliced

sifted icing sugar (optional)

1 Whisk the egg whites until they form stiff but moist-looking peaks. Gradually whisk in the sugars, a teaspoonful at a time, and continue to whisk for 1–2 minutes or until thick and glossy.

2 Mix the cornflour with the vinegar and fold into the meringue. Grease and line a large baking sheet and spoon the meringue on to the sheet in 6 mounds, spreading it into circles about 10 cm (4 inches) across.

3 Bake in a preheated oven, 140°C (275°F), Gas Mark 1, for 35–40 minutes or until crisp on the outside and they can be lifted easily off the paper. Leave to cool.

4 Peel the pavlovas off the paper and transfer them to serving plates. Spoon the crème fraîche over the top and decorate with the berries. To serve, dust with a little sifted icing sugar, if liked.

Nutrition
Wheat free, high fibre
Kcals 109
Fat 2 g
Saturated fat 1 g
Sodium 73 g
Fibre 7 g

Preparation time
10 minutes
Cooking time
none
Serves
4

✚ NUTRITIONAL TIP
To reduce the fibre content, make up
your own bags of fresh strawberries and
raspberries only. Soya yogurt will make
this dessert suitable for a milk-free and
exclusion diet.

cheats' summer berry sundae

This really speedy dessert is made in a matter of seconds and is just bursting
with flavour. Crème de cassis could be used in place of the cordial if you prefer,
and dainty soft amaretti biscuits or biscotti could be served alongside if you are
not avoiding wheat.

**500 g (1 lb) frozen mixed
summer berries, partially
thawed**

**3 tablespoons blackcurrant
cordial (undiluted)**

**250 g (8 oz) low fat Greek
yogurt**

4 teaspoons clear honey

2 tablespoons chopped mint

1 Put the fruit and cordial into a food processor or liquidizer
and blitz until crushed and sorbet like.

2 Mix the yogurt with the honey and chopped mint. Add
alternate spoonfuls of puréed fruit and yogurt to 4 glasses,
then swirl together with the handle of a teaspoon to give a
marbled effect.

3 Decorate with extra mint leaves or a tiny sprig of mint
dusted lightly with sifted icing sugar, if liked.

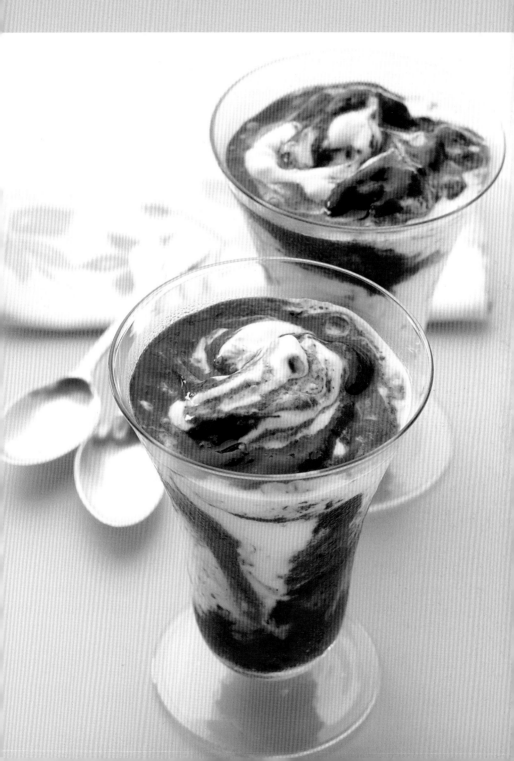

Nutrition

Wheat free, gluten free

Kcals 332

Fat 6 g

Saturated fat 4 g

Sodium 89 mg

Fibre 3 g

Preparation time

20 minutes

Cooking time

40–45 minutes

Serves

4

✚ **NUTRITIONAL TIP**

To reduce the fibre level, use white arborio rice and cook for 20 minutes until tender. To lower the fat levels, use reduced-fat yogurt. For a dairy-free version, use soya milk or rice milk to make the risotto. This will make it suitable for an exclusion diet.

red rice risotto with roasted plums

Spoon down through the hot roasted plums to a generous spoonful of crème fraîche and then into the warmth of the nutty red rice scented with vanilla and cinnamon. Use pitted cherries in season or try stirring a little cocoa powder into the rice along with the sugar for a change.

200 g (7 oz) red rice

450 ml (¾ pint) semi-skimmed milk

450 ml (¾ pint) water

¼ teaspoon ground cinnamon, plus extra to sprinkle

250 g (8 oz) ripe red plums, quartered and pitted

2 tablespoons caster sugar

1 teaspoon vanilla extract

4 tablespoons reduced-fat crème fraîche

1 Put the rice, half the milk and water and the cinnamon into a saucepan. Bring to the boil, reduce the heat and simmer for 40–45 minutes, stirring occasionally and topping up with milk and water as needed until the rice is soft and creamy.

2 Towards the end of the cooking time for the rice, put the plums into a shallow, ovenproof dish, sprinkle with a little extra cinnamon and add a tablespoon of water to the base of the dish. Bake in a preheated oven, 180°C (350F), Gas Mark 4, for 10 minutes.

3 Stir the sugar and vanilla extract into the rice. Spoon into shallow dishes, top with spoonfuls of crème fraîche, sprinkle with a little extra cinnamon and arrange the plums to the side of the crème fraîche.

Nutrition

Wheat, gluten and milk free

Kcals 108

Fat 0 g

Saturated fat 0 g

Sodium 7 mg

Fibre 3 g

Preparation time

10 minutes

Cooking time

15–20 minutes

Serves

4

NUTRITIONAL TIP

If you are not avoiding dairy products, serve the pears with spoonfuls of reduced-fat crème fraîche, Greek yogurt or fromage frais drizzled with a little extra honey. This dish is suitable for an exclusion diet.

saffron and ginger poached pears

Quick and easy to prepare, these light and refreshing poached pears taste just as delicious served warm or chilled. They also freeze well, so why not make up a double quantity in advance of a supper to share with friends?

300 ml (½ pint) apple juice

2 large pinches of saffron threads

1 cm (½ inch) root ginger, peeled and cut into thin strips

1 tablespoon set or clear honey

4 conference pears, each about 150 g (5 oz)

1 Put the apple juice, saffron, ginger and honey into a medium-sized saucepan and heat gently for 5 minutes.

2 Meanwhile, peel the pears, leaving the stalks on, and remove the calyx from the base. Add the pears to the saucepan and press below the surface of the apple juice. (If necessary change to a smaller pan.)

3 Simmer gently for 15–20 minutes, turning the pears from time so that they colour evenly and are just tender. Spoon into a small pedestal dish and serve warm or chilled.

Nutrition
Low fat, gluten free
Kcals 155
Fat 1 g
Saturated fat 0 g
Sodium 16 mg
Fibre 3 g

Preparation time
10 minutes
Cooking time
4–5 minutes
Serves
4

✚ NUTRITIONAL TIP
Anyone on a milk-free or exclusion
diet could use soya yogurt instead
of fromage frais.

maple-glazed pineapple

Speedy enough to prepare while someone else clears the main course plates, this
colourful dessert is just the thing to make for a last-minute meal to share with friends.

**6 slices fresh pineapple, peeled,
cored and halved**

125 g (4 oz) blueberries

8 teaspoons maple syrup

**1 banana, about 200 g (7 oz)
with skin on**

**100 g (3½ oz) low fat fromage
frais**

**2 teaspoons chopped glacé
ginger or stem ginger, drained
and chopped**

1 Arrange the pineapple slices in a single layer on a deep
baking sheet. Sprinkle the blueberries over and around the
pineapple, then drizzle the pineapple with 4 teaspoons
maple syrup.

2 Cook the fruit under a preheated grill for 4–5 minutes until
the pineapple is beginning to brown and the juices have
begun to run from the blueberries.

3 Meanwhile, peel and mash the banana and mix it with the
fromage frais and ginger.

4 Arrange the pineapple on serving plates. Spoon the
blueberries and their juices over the top and the banana
fromage frais to one side. Drizzle with the remaining maple
syrup and serve immediately.

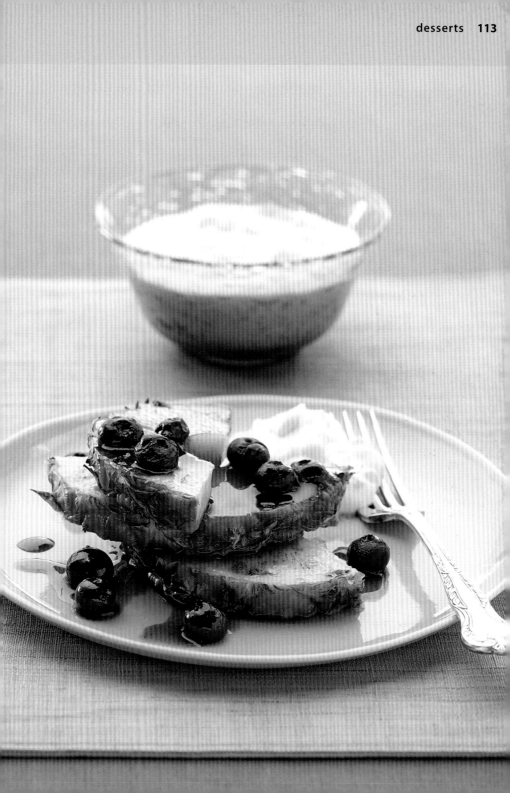

Nutrition

High fibre

Kcals 386

Fat 14 g

Saturated fat 2 g

Sodium 90 mg

Fibre 7 g

Preparation time

20 minutes

Cooking time

25–30 minutes

Serves

4

✚ NUTRITIONAL TIP

If you are avoiding dairy products, use soya margarine and do not serve with custard or ice cream unless made with soya milk. To reduce the fibre content, omit the oats and seeds from the crumble and make up the flour to 100 g (3½ oz).

apple and blackberry flapjack crumble

A homely pudding, this is perfect after a Sunday roast or slow-cooked casserole. The crumble topping can be made in larger batches and kept in the freezer. Simply sprinkle it over cooked fruits while still frozen and transfer to the oven. You might also like to try this with apples only, plums or a mix of plums and pears.

2 cooking apples, about 500 g (1 lb) in total, quartered, cored and peeled

100 g (3½ oz) blackberries

100 g (3½ oz) soft light muscovado sugar

75 g (3 oz) plain flour

50 g (2 oz) reduced-fat spread

40 g (1½ oz) porridge oats

2 tablespoons flaked almonds

2 tablespoons sunflower seeds

finely grated rind of ½ small orange

custard or ice cream, to serve

1 Thinly slice the apples and put them in a saucepan with the blackberries, 2 tablespoons sugar and 6 tablespoons water. Cover and simmer for 5 minutes or until partly cooked.

2 Meanwhile, put the remaining sugar in a bowl with the flour. Add the spread and rub in using your fingertips until the mixture resembles fine breadcrumbs. Stir in the remaining ingredients.

3 Turn the hot fruit into a 900 ml (1½ pint) ovenproof dish, spoon the crumble mixture over the top and bake in a preheated oven, 180°C (350°F), Gas Mark 4, for 25–30 minutes or until golden-brown. Serve with custard or ice cream.

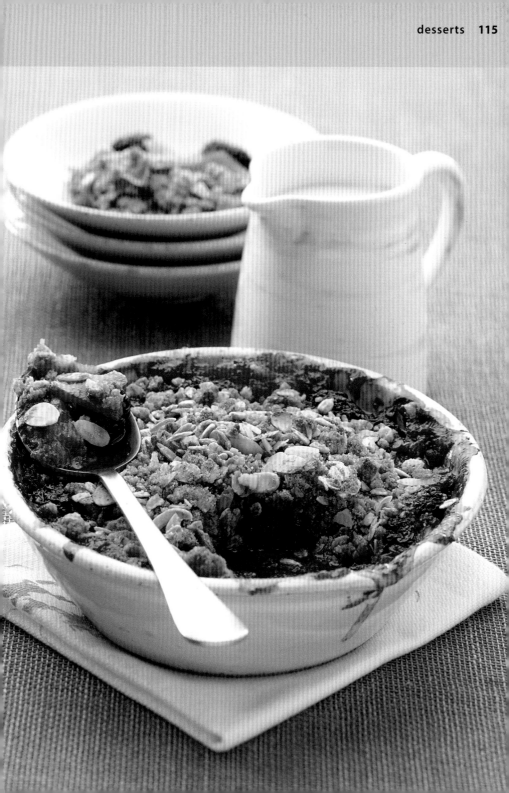

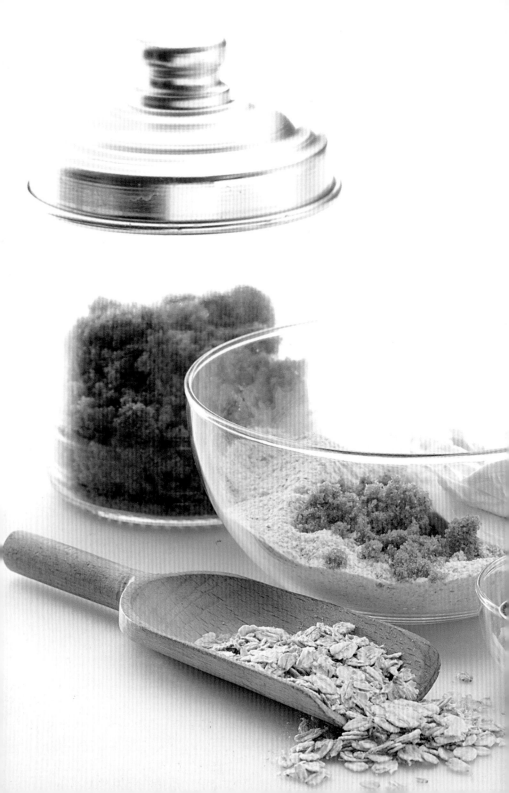

cakes and
bakes

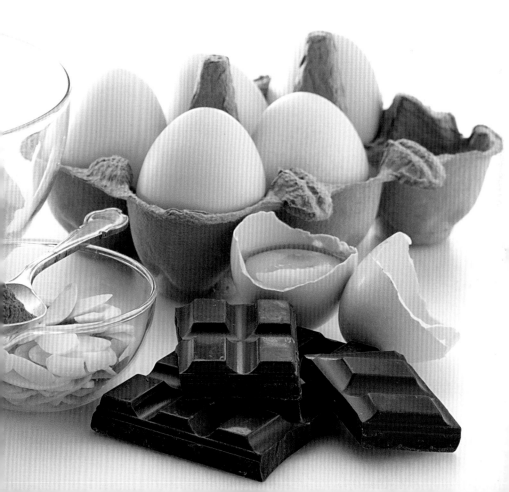

Nutrition

Wheat free, gluten free

Kcals 327

Fat 14 g

Saturated fat 1 g

Sodium 166 mg

Fibre 3 g

Preparation time

30 minutes, plus

cooling

Cooking time

15 minutes

Serves

8

NUTRITIONAL TIP

If you are allergic to nuts but not wheat or gluten, then fold in 100 g (3½ oz) sifted plain flour instead. Check the tinned cherries and cream cheese are gluten free.

cherry and orange roulade

Just because you may be intolerant to wheat flour doesn't mean that you must avoid cakes. This wheat-free roulade uses ground almonds instead.

5 large eggs, separated

250 g (8 oz) caster sugar, plus extra for dusting

100 g (3½ oz) ground almonds

grated rind of 1½ oranges

40 g (1½ oz) flaked almonds

300 g (10 oz) low-fat cream cheese

425 g (14 oz) can stoned cherries, drained

a few fresh cherries (optional)

1 Put the egg yolks and 175 g (6 oz) sugar in a large bowl set over a saucepan of simmering water. Whisk until light and pale. Take the bowl off the saucepan and gently fold in the ground almonds and the rind from 1 orange.

2 Put the egg whites in a separate bowl and whisk until stiff, moist-looking peaks form. Fold a large spoonful into the yolk mixture to loosen it slightly, then gently fold in the rest.

3 Grease and line a 23 x 30 cm (9 x 12 inch) baking tin with a piece of nonstick baking paper. Make diagonal cuts into the corners of the paper, then press it into the tin. Pour in the mixture and ease it into the corners. Sprinkle with the flaked almonds and bake in a preheated oven, 180°F (350°F), Gas Mark 4, for 15 minutes until the roulade is well risen and the top feels spongy. Remove from the oven and leave to cool.

4 Beat the cream cheese with the remaining orange rind and half the remaining sugar. Put a large piece of baking paper on the work surface, dust it with the remaining caster sugar and turn the roulade out on it. Remove the lining paper.

5 Spread the cream cheese mixture over the top, then sprinkle with the cherries. Roll up the roulade, starting from the short edge, using the paper to help. Transfer to a serving plate, remove the paper and cut into thick slices to serve.

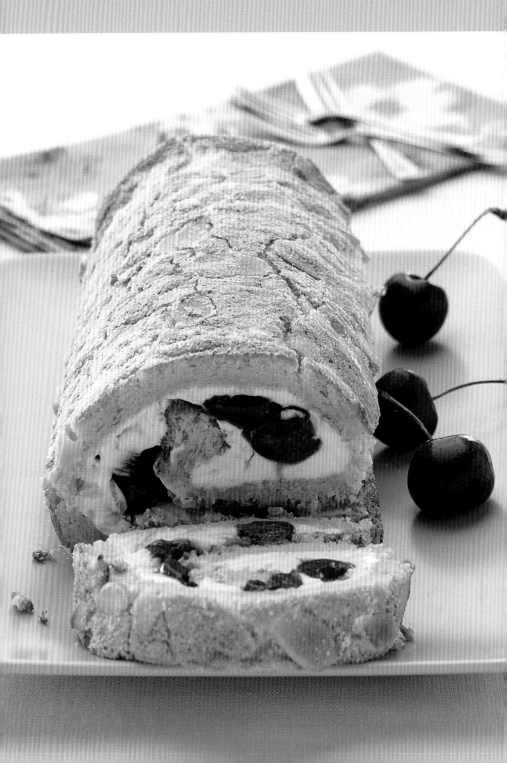

Nutrition

Low fibre

Kcals 66

Fat 3 g

Saturated fat 1 g

Sodium 69 mg

Fibre 1 g

Preparation time

20 minutes

Cooking time

10 minutes

Makes

24 biscuits

NUTRITIONAL TIP

For a dairy-free version, use soya margarine and unsweetened soya milk instead of the low-fat spread and dairy milk. You will also need to omit the chocolate topping.

chocolate cinnamon digestives

Lower in fat and higher in fibre than most shop-bought biscuits, these crumbly biscuits are drizzled with a little chocolate for those moments when you crave something sweet.

175 g (6 oz) wholemeal flour

2 teaspoons baking powder

1 teaspoon ground cinnamon

50 g (2 oz) medium oatmeal

100 g (3½ oz) reduced-fat spread

40 g (1½ oz) soft dark muscovado sugar

3 tablespoons semi-skimmed milk

50 g (2 oz) dark chocolate

1 Put the flour, baking powder, cinnamon and oatmeal into a bowl. Add the spread and rub in with fingertips until the mixture resembles fine breadcrumbs.

2 Stir in the sugar, add the milk and mix to a soft but not sticky dough.

3 Knead lightly, then roll out on a lightly floured surface to 5 mm (¼ inch) thick. Cut out 6 cm (2½ inch) rounds with a fluted or plain biscuit cutter. Transfer the biscuits to an oiled baking sheet, then knead and re-roll the trimmings until all the mixture is used. Prick the biscuits with a fork, then bake in a preheated oven, 200°C (400°F), Gas Mark 6, for 10 minutes or until browned. Leave to cool.

4 Melt the chocolate in a bowl set over a pan of gently simmering water. Drizzle or pipe squiggly lines of chocolate from a spoon over the top of the biscuits. Leave to harden for 20 minutes, then serve. The biscuits will keep for up to 5 days in an airtight tin.

Nutrition

Dairy free

Kcals 194

Fat 7 g

Saturated fat 2 g

Sodium 157 mg

Fibre 3 g

Preparation time

25 minutes

Cooking time

30–35 minutes

Makes

16 squares

NUTRITIONAL TIP

To lower the level of fibre, use white flour rather than a mix of white and brown and omit the seeds on top. If you are not avoiding dairy products, use reduced-fat spread and semi-skimmed cows' milk instead of the soya products.

banana and fig gingerbread

This moist, golden gingerbread is flecked with naturally sweet bananas and chopped dried figs, so that only syrup has been added to the cake rather than the more usual mix of syrup and sugar. This cake keeps well in an airtight tin, so is ideal for adding to packed lunchboxes.

100 g (3½ oz) soya margarine

175 g (6 oz) golden syrup

150 g (5 oz) figs, chopped

150 ml (¼ pint) unsweetened soya milk

2 tablespoons chopped glacé ginger

125 g (4 oz) self-raising flour

125 g (4 oz) plain wholemeal flour

3 teaspoons ground ginger

1 teaspoon bicarbonate of soda

2 ripe bananas, about 175 g (6 oz) each with their skins on, peeled and mashed

2 eggs, beaten

2 tablespoons sunflower seeds (optional)

1 Put the margarine, syrup, figs, milk and ginger in a saucepan and heat gently until the margarine has melted.

2 Mix all the dry ingredients together in a bowl. Beat the eggs in a second small bowl.

3 Take the saucepan off the heat, then mix in the bananas and dry ingredients with a wooden spoon. Gradually beat in the eggs.

4 Grease and line a 20 cm (8 inch) square cake tin and pour the mixture into the tin. Sprinkle with the seeds (if used) and bake in a preheated oven, 180°C (350°F), Gas Mark 4, for 30–35 minutes until the cake is well risen and the top springs back when pressed with a fingertip. Leave the cake to cool in the tin.

5 Remove from the tin, peel off the lining paper and cut into 16 squares. Store in an airtight tin for up to 7 days.

Nutrition
Wheat and gluten free, low fibre
Kcals 380
Fat 21 g
Saturated fat 11 g
Sodium 82 g
Fibre 2 g

Preparation time
40 minutes, plus
cooling
Cooking time
15–18 minutes
Serves
8

Nutritional tip
Choose chocolate that is 70 per cent
cocoa solids, as it should be completely
wheat free and gluten free, but always
check the label.

chocolate and raspberry layer cake

This wheat-free cake is perfect for a birthday celebration. Alternatively, serve it as a dessert with a drizzle of puréed raspberry sauce (see page 104). The cakes can be frozen on their own or fully assembled with the raspberries and chocolate curls.

200 g (7 oz) plain dark chocolate, chopped

6 eggs, separated

175 g (6 oz) caster sugar, plus extra for dusting

2 tablespoons warm water

150 ml (¼ pint) whipping cream

150 g (5 oz) Greek yogurt

250 g (8 oz) raspberries

chocolate curls, to decorate

1 Put the chocolate in a bowl set over a saucepan of gently simmering water and leave for 5 minutes until melted.

2 Lift the chocolate bowl off the pan, set a second large bowl on top of the water, add the egg yolks and sugar and whisk for 5 minutes until very light and pale and the whisk leaves a trail when lifted out of the mixture. Take the bowl off the pan and gently fold in the chocolate and measured warm water.

3 In a clean bowl whisk the egg white until stiff but moist-looking peaks form. Fold a large spoonful into the yolks mixture to loosen it, then fold in the remainder.

4 Grease and line 2 round 20 cm (8 inch) sandwich tins and divide the mixture equally between them. Bake in a preheated oven, 180°C (350°F), Gas Mark 4, for 15–18 minutes until well risen and the tops are crusty and cracked and softly set in the centre. Remove from the oven. Leave to cool in the tins.

5 Whip the cream until it holds its shape, then fold in the yogurt. Turn out the cakes and put one on a serving plate. Top with half the cream mixture and half the raspberries. Add the second cake, the remaining cream and raspberries and then complete with a few chocolate curls. Cut into slices to serve.

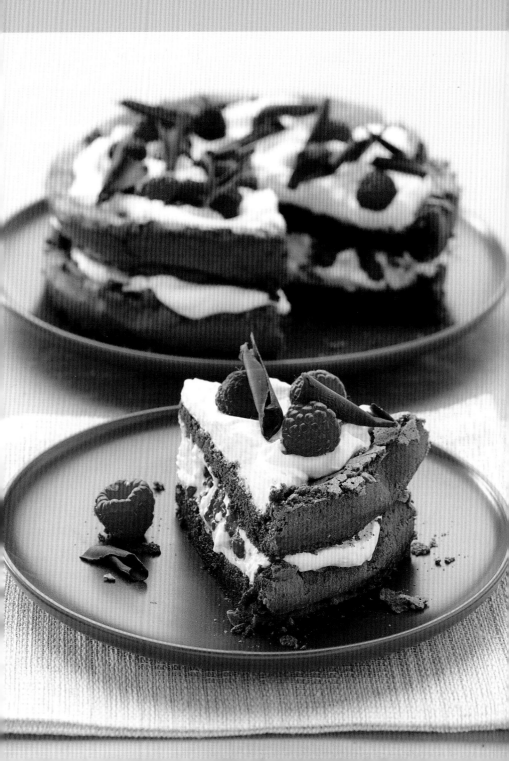

Nutrition
Wheat and gluten free, low fibre
Kcals 323
Fat 11 g
Saturated fat 3 g
Sodium 164 mg
Fibre 2 g

Preparation time
30 minutes
Cooking time
30–35 minutes
Serves
8

NUTRITIONAL TIP
White flour can be used if you are not on a wheat- or gluten-free diet. Use soya margarine to make this cake suitable for a dairy-free diet.

apple sauce cake

No one will guess that this cake is wheat free. Serve while it's still warm on its own or with a spoonful of reduced-fat crème fraîche or soya yogurt for a dairy-free alternative. Drizzled with custard, it doubles as a pudding.

2 cooking apples, each about 250 g (8 oz), cored, peeled and thinly sliced

little lemon juice

250 g (8 oz) wheat- and gluten-free white bread flour with natural gum

2½ teaspoons wheat- and gluten-free baking powder

1 teaspoon ground cinnamon

½ teaspoon ground ginger

¼ teaspoon grated nutmeg

3 eggs

150 g (5 oz) reduced-fat spread

175 g (6 oz) caster sugar

1 Put half the apple slices in a small saucepan with 2 tablespoons water, then cover and simmer for 5 minutes until pulpy. Put the remaining apple slices in a bowl of cold water with a little lemon juice.

2 Mix the flour, baking powder, half the cinnamon and all the ginger and nutmeg together in a second bowl. Beat the eggs in a jug.

3 Cream the reduced-fat spread with 150 g (5 oz) sugar in a bowl. Gradually mix in alternate spoonfuls of egg and flour mix to the creamed mixture until both have been added and the mixture is smooth. Stir in the cooked apple.

4 Pour the mixture into a lightly oiled 23 cm (9 inch) spring-form cake tin and smooth the top. Drain the remaining apples well and arrange the slices in rings on top of the cake mixture. Sprinkle with the remaining sugar and cinnamon. Bake in a preheated oven, 180°C (350°F), Gas Mark 4, for 35–40 minutes until well risen and a skewer inserted into the centre of the cake comes out cleanly.

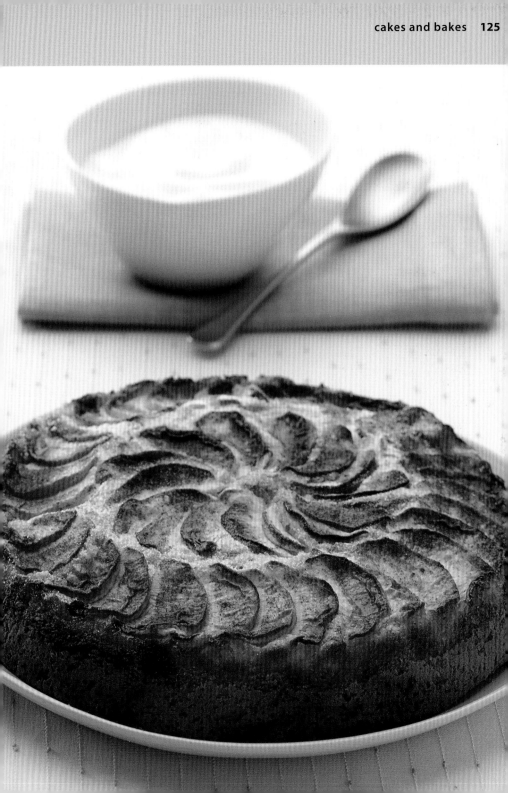

index

USEFUL CONTACTS

Britain

IBS Network
Helpline: 0114 272 3253
www.ibsnetwork.org.uk
A national charity, providing the only dedicated support in the UK to people with IBS, helping them and their families and carers to manage their IBS and achieve an improved quality of life. For the fact sheet 'IBS Information and Advice' send a SAE to the above address.

Allergy UK
Helpline: 01322 619898
www.allergyuk.org

British Dietetic Association
www.bda.uk.com
Access to an informative fact sheet on a range of diet-related issues written by registered dieticians on their website.

British Society of Medical and Dental Hypnosis
Tel: 07000 560 309
www.bsmdh.org
To search for a health professional with expertise in hypnotherapy.

Dieticians Unlimited
www.dieticiansunlimited.co.uk
To search for a dietician with expertise in IBS via their website.

Health Professions Council (HPC)
Tel: 020 7582 0866
www.hpc-uk.org
Check your dietician is registered by logging on to the HPC website.

Australia

Irritable Bowel Information and Support Association of Australia (IBIS Australia)
Tel: 0061 (0)7 3907 0527
www.ibis-australia.org

Dietitians Association of Australia (DAA)
Tel: 0061 (0)2 6282 9555
www.daa.asn.au
You can find an Accredited Practising Dietician (APD) who has expertise in treating IBS.

Canada

IBS Association
www.ibsassociation.org

USA

IBS Association (IBSA)
www.ibsassociation.org

IBS Self-help Group (IBS Group)
www.ibsgroup.org

American Dietetic Association
www.eatright.org
Tel: 001 800 877 1600
You can find a registered nutrition professional with expertise in IBS through this site.

ACKNOWLEDGEMENTS

Tracy Parker would like to thank Alex Riordan BSc (Hons) RD, Dr David Preston, Dr Ed Stoner and Helen Francis for their helpful comments and advice.

Executive editor: Nicola Hill
Editor: Camilla Davis
Executive art editor:
        Darren Southern
Home economist: Sara Lewis
Designer: Colin Goody
Picture research: Jennifer Veall
Production: Nigel Reed

PICTURE CREDITS